Lori S. Wiener

50

Pathological Play in Borderline and Narcissistic Personalities

Pathological Play in Borderline and Narcissistic Personalities

Patterns of Real and Not-Real Meaning in Splitting and Denial; Love, Hate, and Ambivalence; and Social Ideology

IRVING STEINGART, PH.D.

Clinical Professor of Psychology
New York University
Post Doctoral Program in Psychotherapy and Psychoanalysis

SP

SP MEDICAL & SCIENTIFIC BOOKS
a division of Spectrum Publications, Inc.
New York

SPECTRUM PUBLICATIONS, INC.
175-20 Wexford Terrace, Jamaica, N.Y. 11432

Library of Congress Cataloging in Publication Data

Steingart, Irving.
Pathological play in borderline-narcissistic personalities.

Includes index.
1. Personality, Disorders of. 2. Cognition.
3. Narcissism. I. Title. [DNLM: 1. Narcissism.
2. Cognition. WM 460.5.E3 S882c]
RC554.S73 616.89 82-3281
ISBN 0-89335-179-2

For (in order of appearance) Joyce, Amy, and David

Foreword

In recent years, Otto Kernberg, in forcefully propounding the "borderline personality organization" as a discrete diagnostic entity, has brought a significant debate to the forefront of psychoanalysis. Pithily described by Arnold Cooper as the debate between "lumpers" and "splitters," the opponents in this controversy are, respectively, those analysts who "lump," i.e., who view psychopathology along a continuum in which the differences between different diagnostic categories are quantitative rather than qualitative, and those analysts who "split," i.e., who believe that qualitative differences exist between the neurotic, borderline, and psychotic diagnostic groupings. To this timely dialogue within our profession, the present study of Irving Steingart constitutes a valuable contribution. Nominally a "splitter," Steingart undertakes the ambitious task of defining a special type of borderline reality testing disturbance. In positing a connection between borderline disturbance and a specific type of cognitive defect, he offers us a closely reasoned and meticulously researched consideration of borderline phenomena from the standpoint of child development, cognitive psychology (Piaget, Werner, Kaplan), and psychoanalysis. Steingart's contribution is to be especially welcomed by virtue of its erudite integration of a cognitive (Piagetian) vantage point with affective considerations framed within Freudian metapsychology. As the outcome of his inquiry, Steingart emerges with three provocative new concepts which, he believes, are integral to borderline phenomena: those of a "meaning disturbance," of "pathological play," and of "paradoxical creation." By fusing Piaget's insights into the formation of the child's sense of meaning with psychoanalytic insights bearing on the formation of intrapsychic structures, the repetition-compulsion, and the role of ambivalence, Steingart's work offers the prospect of a much needed affective-cognitive integration in our overall approach to borderline disturbance.

Steingart's constructs should prove valuable to our understanding of adult borderline pathology because they derive from important insights about early cognitive development. In the past, it has proven extremely difficult if not impossible to substantiate constructs of this sort with analytic data gathered from clinical work with adults. To its credit, Steingart's major hypothesis, in view of its specificity, may ultimately prove testable clinically and perhaps even experimentally. It may indeed be possible, that is, to demonstrate cognitive differences between groups of patients diagnosed as borderline and nonborderline. Such differences would pertain to the measurable degree of "borderline pathology" which Steingart understands as the ability to differentiate between "real" and "not real" experience. Whether or not differences of this sort can in fact be demonstrated, Steingart's clarifying, testable propositions, teamed with his integrative cognitive-analytic perspective on the genesis of borderline pathology in general, can only advance our understanding of patients with such disturbances.

Having perhaps too summarily classified Steingart as a "splitter" with respect to his conceptualization of borderline phenomena, I should add at once that I perceive him as a splitter with a difference. When he discusses psychic development, that is, he adopts a point of view that goes well beyond a simple dichotomy of borderline and nonborderline phenomena. Steingart knows fully well that "it is the task of developmental psychoanalytic psychology to document theoretically both emergent change and continuity in the life cycle," and he emphasizes throughout that the concepts of differentiation and development are equally central to a psychoanalytic conceptualization of development.*

It is instructive to consider briefly just how Steingart's developmental assumptions relate to several further controversies within psychoanalysis. In the course of propounding his interactive perspective on development, he does not see fit (like Gill, Schafer, and others) to jettison the structural agencies of id, ego, and superego; rather, he adopts the reasonable viewpoint that "if we did not have our id, ego, and superego psychic systems concepts, we would have to invent some others to perform this theoretical task for us." Correspondingly, he is critical of those analysts who supplant the structural agencies with "self" concepts in the hope of rendering analysis more experientially immediate to the clinical concerns of patients. Such analysts, for Steingart, labor under a "confusion between what is meant by immediate experience and what we mean by psychic content in psychoanalysis." It follows that Steingart sharply disagrees with Kohut's contention that a "psychology of the self" is necessary to deal with the problems of narcissism. For Steingart, Kohut's theorizing actually reflects a failure to distinguish between psychic content and the structure of the psychic apparatus itself. His own position, with which I am in agreement, is that content and structure are discrete yet interactively connected dimensions of mental life. They are analogous to the way in which the software (content) and hardware (structure) of a computer are, in Steingart's own words, "ingredients of the same computer." Finally, with respect to the continuing debate about the status of

---

*In this respect, Steingart's perspective is akin to that of Feffer in his recent work, *The Structure of Freudian Thought* (1982). Feffer discusses the problem of "immutability and discontinuity" in development theory. His thesis is that this problem has not been adequately solved by psychoanalysis and, like Steingart, he invokes Piaget in attempting to resolve the paradox.

psychoanalysis as a hermeneutic or a natural-scientific enterprise, Steingart successfully avoids falling into a self-limiting either-or dichotomy. His notion of a "meaning apparatus" captures, I believe, his sound understanding of the fact that antithetical concepts are intrinsic to the psychoanalytic endeavor; neither the hermeneutic nor the natural-scientific viewpoint can be ignored if our conceptualizations are to be fully adequate.

Beyond its contribution to these general controversies, Steingart's work contributes to a more specific debate focusing on the status of "splitting" as a major defense implicated in borderline conditions. The terms of this debate have been set by Kernberg, who has argued in recent years that borderline patients utilize the pathognomic primitive defenses of splitting and projective identification, and that these defenses take shape during the first 18 months of life. The Kris Study Group on Borderline Patients, it should be noted, has taken partial exception to Kernberg's position in arguing that these defenses, and the distorted object relations associated with them, cannot be attributed to a specific early stage of ego development. In Steingart's case, Kernberg's attribution of specificity with respect to the early phase of development at which splitting occurs would be translated into an attribution of specificity with respect to the early cognitive stage in which borderline disturbances are rooted and, to this degree, he ostensibly sides with Kernberg in this dispute. Beyond the matter of the point in development at which splitting occurs, there is the related issue of just how such splitting is to be construed. Steingart, with Kernberg, would view such splitting as a "primitive defense" which reflects developmental failure in early life. Steingart defines splitting as "consciousness mediated by repetition compulsion in an area of immature meaning structure, function and content." The Kris Study Group on Borderline Patients (Abend et al., in press), for its part, conceptualizes splitting, along with other early defenses (idealization, omnipotence, devaluation), as complex derivatives of unconscious fantasies to be understood in terms of the total organization of the ego. In linking splitting to unconscious fantasies, of course, the Study Group clearly departs from the major emphasis of Kernberg and Steingart; in situating such fantasies within a conception of the total organization of the ego, however, the Group's perspective seemingly allows for the type of developmental cognitive disturbance with which Steingart is concerned.

On a different point, there is clinical agreement between Kernberg and the members of the Kris Study Group. Both believe that borderline patients are marked by a relative inability to accept the "as if" quality of their transference wishes and fears and by an associated need for literal gratifications from their analysts. It is perhaps with reference to this area of clinical consensus that Steingart's cognitive-analytic perspective is most germane, offering as it does both a formulation and an explanation of this clinical state of affairs. The outstanding question, of course, is whether such transference phenomena are to be understood as a consequence of ego defect or a defective self-observing capacity which may, to be sure, be implicated in psychic conflict, or whether, in the spirit of the Kris Study Group, they routinely reflect a failure of reality testing that is linked to a complex interplay of defenses against anxiety, guilt, and other unpleasurable affects.

In summary, I believe Steingart has made an original contribution to the issue of borderline diagnosis that simultaneously constitutes a significant commentary on several timely debates within psychoanalysis, including the role of the "self" in psychoanalytic theory and the status of psychoanalysis as a hermeneutic or a natural-scientific enterprise. With respect to the issue of the self, Steingart does not follow theorists like Kohut, Gedo, and G. Klein in elevating the self to a superordinate conceptual status. Rather, he is concerned throughout with the development of self and object representations and with disturbances related to conflict in the realm of self representation. His focus on "real" and "not real" self experience keeps his conceptualizations at that experiential level which is most relevant to clinical work. Of special note is his interesting elucidation of the concept of play; he believes that play evokes childhood experiences of make-believe, dress-up, and similar activities in which self and identity are explored and their respective boundaries delimited. It remains for psychoanalytic clinicians to incorporate Steingart's provocative concepts into their theoretical armamentarium and to report on their clinical usefulness. In particular, it remains to be seen whether clinical experience will bear out his central hypothesis about a specific cognitive disturbance associated with borderline pathology. In any event, Steingart's cogent, scholarly presentation of his case makes it imperative that his hypothesis be seriously entertained. His book certainly deserves a careful reading by psychoanalytic theorist and clinician alike.

Arnold Richards, M.D.

References

Abend S., Porder M., and Willick M. Monograph of the Kris Study Group: *Psychoanalytic Perspectives on the Borderline Patient.* International Universities Press (in press).

Preface

It occurs in our literature that if one considers something about cognition, and then how this cognitive consideration can relate to other, more usual psychoanalytic conceptualizations (dynamics, object relations, narcissism, whatever), this cognitive consideration then can be given a kind of status which works against a fruitful integration. It is like an unwholesome idealization that interferes with a healthy love or work relationship. The cognitive consideration is treated as if it were some special, honored guest invited into a home with whom the family cannot be entirely comfortable about being itself, and therefore cannot be natural. On the other hand, it also certainly occurs in our literature that a cognitive consideration is treated as if it were some distant relative whose personal characteristics and customs are not felt to be congenial, or good enough, for the familial way of life. I hope that neither of these two outcomes is the result of the cognitive considerations I describe in this book. One does not have to belabor the fact that cognitive processes are, and always have been, intimate members of that conceptual family which has the name psychoanalytic theory. Freud (1895 [1950a]) devoted a good deal of the Project to cognitive considerations. Cognitive processes are the subject matter of the famous Chapter Seven in the dream book (Freud, 1900a), and one easily can find Freud's interest in one or the other aspect of cognition in many other places in his writing. Cognitive considerations should enjoy easy—which means mutually constitutive—relations with all other aspects of psychoanalytic theory. This is the spirit with which I have written this book.

How could it be otherwise? Suppose, starting now, each of us began to realize that we were learning to fly. We began to notice as we jogged, or as we ran for a train, that we were lifting off the ground, and we sensed what we had to do to stay aloft. Suppose all of us, then, learned to fly. Can anyone doubt the extraordinary significance that this capability for flying would have for the meaning of our existence? In fact, an equally startling and significant capability actually occurs in our development when each of us changes from crawling to upright locomotion. Most of us have become jaded to this experience. Not so the young child. The toddler is euphoric about himself or herself when upright locomotion is accomplished (e.g., Mahler, Pine, and Bergman, 1975). We celebrate this momentous achievement with the sports of track and field.

However, my interest now is not in locomotion but in the capability for thinking—representation. And my point is that each of us experiences an equally extraordinary change in the nature of our existence when we acquire a capability for representation. Equally extraordinary changes occur in how we feel and know our existence which relate to emergent changes in this capability for representation. Most of us also have been jaded to these spectacular events with, I believe, a consequent loss for our theory. We, like birds, do take to flight with the development of our capability for thought. To say that this thinking apparatus (Hartmann, 1939), its emergent characteristics with development, has no ongoing, intimate relationship with the deep subject matter of psychoanalysis is like saying that the fact that a bird can fly is not a terribly important feature of every other aspect of the bird's life. Something I believed to be important about how cognition participates in personality (dis)organization already was described by me in a 1969 paper entitled "On Self, Character, and Development of a Psychic Apparatus." This book represents a much more complete realization of those ideas, which come out of two sources.

First and foremost, there are my personal analyses, and also my work as a psychoanalyst and therapist with adults and children; and allied to this work is my work as a supervisor and teacher, which always hold one's conceptual tools up to the light. Some further development of my ideas became part of a course I taught during the spring in the years 1974 and 1975 at the New York University Postdoctoral Program, entitled "Aspects of Character Formation."

The second work source is research and teaching done by me at Downstate Medical Center during the years 1967 to 1977. While at Downstate I worked as a member of the Clinical Behavior Research Unit. The Research Unit's interest was communication behavior, or better stated, what vicissitudes in communication behavior could reveal about (dis)organization of personality. My particular responsibility was to familiarize myself with linguistic and psycholinguistic literature and to develop language communication measures pertinent to the overall purpose of the Research Unit. It also became my responsibility, while at Downstate, to teach in the Doctor of Medical Science Program. This is a program designed for a psychiatrist who wishes to acquire knowledge and skills about how to conduct psychological research. Certain courses in this Doctor of Medical Science Program also were used by Fellows in Child Psychiatry at Downstate, and one such course was a course I taught in the fall of 1974 and 1976, entitled "Language, Cognition, and Character Formation." As is obvious from the title of this course, its subject matter was the interpenetration of cognitive matters with personality. This course afforded me an opportunity to think about this subject matter. But, as well, the course required me always to explicate the relevance of whatever such ideas I had to clinical practice, especially inasmuch as the large part of the student body always was composed of Fellows in training to become child psychiatrists. I freely "tinkered" with the contents of this course, according to what seemed new and important to me, and I was given a completely free hand to do this by Dr. Adolph Christ, Head of Child Psychiatry at Downstate. I am grateful to Dr. Christ for his generous assumption that whatever changes in content I deemed worthwhile would turn out to have relevance for the training of his Fellows in Child Psychiatry. Dr. Norbert Freedman is Director of the Doctor in Medical Science Program, Dr. Stanley Grand is the Program's Associate Director, and it is especially with these two individuals as research colleagues that I conducted research into language behavior.

Notwithstanding some important changes I made in my work schedule, to free up time to write this book, there was not enough time. Time needed to be spent at home. My wish to write this book had to be worked through with my family, and this makes the writing of the book an even more important achievement for me. I want to thank my wife, Joyce Steingart, for both her professional expertise and critical examination of the manuscript, as well as her personal support. I want to thank my children, Amy and David, for their support and encouragement. The subject matter of this book is arranged developmentally. What development means to me is in a special way alive because I have children, and this, of course, means that David and Amy participate in my development.

Another group of people to whom I am especially indebted are the members of my study group, each of whom read an entire draft of the manuscript and provided me with numerous useful comments. These people are Sheldon Bach, Norbert Freedman, Mark Grunes, and Martin Nass. We not only study but also go through life together.

Steven Ellman, Donald Kaplan, Stanley Grand, and Arnold Richards, also read an entire draft of the manuscript and made helpful comments.

Esther Menaker and Leo Goldberger were especially supportive and helpful to me in my efforts to get this book a publisher.

I want to express my appreciation to Henny Ostrower and Nina Kimche, who typed earlier drafts of parts of the manuscript, and to Alexa Pierce, who typed an entire earlier draft. All these typists showed not only forebearance but a saving intelligence in the face of transcription machinery which was far from the best and copy which could take on an uncomfortable resemblance to the production of a neophyte Boy Scout first learning how to mark out some trail in the woods.

Joann Kirtland, besides typing the final draft, first afforded me superb editorial assistance with the organization and logic of the manuscript, and I am grateful to her.

Finally, I want to return to the beginning of these remarks. Initially, I spoke about a desire that the cognitive considerations raised in this book be recognized as a true family member of that conceptual entirety we designate as psychoanalytic theory. I do not want to hide from an implication that this metaphor has for psychoanalytic theory. In a family which is anywhere near something psychologically viable, influence from each member must show somehow in family life. In other words, and to change metaphors, I do believe that the cognitive considerations I describe in this book do call for a change, but one in what we might consider to be the center of gravity of psychoanalytic theory. The center of gravity, wherever it is located, always reflects the influences of all aspects of a system. I believe all of the conceptual reorientations wrought upon psychoanalytic theory—the structural approach initiated by Freud himself (1923b), the object relations viewpoint (e.g., Kernberg, 1975a), a perspective which emphasizes a narcissistic line of development (e.g., Kohut, 1977), etc.—all should be viewed as effecting a change in the location of the centering of psychoanalytic theory. And of course all such change in the design of the theory was a response to serious issues met with in our work. With respect to what I call in this book the meaning apparatus perspective, I think it first was our work with children which inclined psychoanalytic theory to appreciate such an influence. More recently, I believe that the not-typical—that is to say, other-than-neurotic—transference formats shown by borderline and narcissistic individuals ought to contribute to an appreciation of such an influence. But whatever the change in theoretical centering which may be wrought upon psychoanalysis, Freudian psychoanalysis still remains Freudian psychoanalysis. A car may be redesigned to have a lower center of gravity in order to effect a better grip on road turns, but it is still a car.

I end with a final metaphor, an old and familiar one, and stated more personally. If, as I believe, a certain cognitive perspective enables us to see borderline and narcissistic phenomena better, it is because it already sits upon other, hard-won, important psychoanalytic conceptualization. It is like a boy who is boosted upon his father's shoulders so that the boy actually can come to see more than the father himself. This is a very natural development for the two of them.

Contents

The imagination of a boy is healthy, and the mature imagination of a man is healthy; but there is a space of life between, in which the soul is in a ferment, the character undecided, the way of life uncertain, the ambition thicksighted: thence proceeds mawkishness, and the thousand bitters which those men I speak of must necessarily taste in going over the following pages.

John Keats
(Preface to *Endymion*)

Love is anterior to life,
Posterior to death,
Initial of creation, and
The exponent of breath.

Emily Dickinson

I tell you there is such a thing as creative hate!

Willa Sibert Cather
(*The Song of the Lark*)

1
Introduction

There is something amusing, as well as serious, about the change in our psychoanalytic literature with regards to the concept of "borderline." It is as if a family in some small, closely knit town, which had had some checkered past in its origins, now had achieved not only widespread acceptance, but also status in the community; whereas earlier this family and its supporters were a beleaguered minority, they are now an overwhelming majority, and the now minority dissenters are regarded as backward purists.

In an article written thirty years ago, Robert Knight (1953) began with the following sentence: "The term 'borderline state' has achieved almost no official status in psychiatric nomenclature, and conveys no diagnostic illumination of a case other than the implication that a patient is quite sick but not frankly psychotic" (p. 1). Knight goes on to cite comments by authorities such as Rickman (1928), Glover (1932), and Zilboorg (1941), all of whom regarded the term "borderline" as a kind of undesireable "escape hatch," something used by an analyst to relieve his or her clinical and consequently conceptual frustration in working with a certain individual. I believe that this still remains a serious consideration in the application of the term "borderline" to any particular person with whom we work in therapy and with whom our work is very difficult. Now, almost thirty years later, the term "borderline" is still the subject of hot debate. But certainly now the entire conceptual climate has changed.

However, for all this change in conceptual climate, this "checkered past" does not simply go away. Knight (1953) commented that he had no wish "to defend the term 'borderline state'" (p. 2) and wanted in his article only to give a thoughtful, careful description of the "functional psychiatric conditions" (p. 2) for which the term "borderline" is applied. But careful description aside, the gist of Knight's (1953) conception of borderline nevertheless is evident, and this is that "it is quite possible for both psychotic and neurotic mechanisms to have developed in the same individual, and this is the crux of the problem in many borderline cases" (p. 4). What naturally goes along with this are certain other ideas. For example, a "break with reality. . .must be thought of not as a sudden and unexpected snapping, as of a twig, but as a *gradual bending* as well" (p. 3, italics mine); and "the aim should be to take a complete inventory of ego functioning in order to discover the kind of equilibrium which exists between ego controls on the one hand and threatening impulses on the other, and to learn whether the *movement* in this patient is toward less ego control and poorer adaptation" (p. 9). I select these quotations (others could be cited) because they point up a matter which remains problematic and which simply will not go away in connection with this concept of borderline. First, there is a question about the status of reality testing for such individuals. Is there actually a way of formulating a qualitatively different type of borderline reality testing which marks it as neither neurotic nor schizophrenic? Clearly, Knight (1953) did not think so, and instead emphasized a roughly quantitative matter of degree of reality testing with his metaphor of a bending twig. The second question is really like the first, only cast in a more general form. Is there actually a way of formulating a qualitatively different type of borderline personality organization which is neither neurotic nor schizophrenic? Again Knight (1953) did not think so, and this is evident when he emphasized how it is important to gauge diagnostically the overall movement of such an individual toward at least neurotic adjustment or away from this towards schizophrenia.

The same questions are still raised. Inasmuch as it is Kernberg (e.g., 1975a) who especially has transformed our conceptual landscape with his conception of the borderline personality, it is to Kernberg that such questions are raised. Calef and Weinshel (1979), in what is overall a harshly critical review, repeatedly come back to what they believe to be, at best, ambiguity, and at worst, contradiction in Kernberg's writings about the borderline personality. Calef and Weinshel (1979) state:

> A particularly illuminating example of this kind of mental acrobatics which Kernberg is obliged to employ in order to defend the essential discreteness of the borderline personality organization as a stable and specific psychological entity can be seen in his attempts to characterize the quality of reality testing in that "condition." (p. 481)

Calef and Weinshel (1979) point out how Kernberg (1975a) states that borderline individuals usually "maintain their capacity for reality testing, *except* under these special circumstances—severe stress, regression induced by alcohol and drugs, and a transference psychosis" (p. 4, italics by Calef and Weinshel). And Calef and Weinshel (1979) respond, "Would we not at least grant the possibility of some measure of impaired reality testing under these circumstances in the widest array of personality organizations from the more fragile psychotics to the reasonably well put together individuals who fall into Kernberg's category of 'high-level character neurosis'?" (p. 481)

Again Kernberg (1975a) states that "frequency and intensity of temporary loss of reality testing are not, themselves, important prognostic indicators" (p. 136). Calef and Weinshel (1979) then point out how a moment later Kernberg

(1975a) talks about "reality testing . . . to the extent to which the individual is aware of his interpersonal or social reality, and especially the moral values of others. . . . Reality testing in this broad sense does have some prognostic value" (p. 137). Or again, Kernberg (1975a) states that "this conceptualization of reality testing is a restricted, delimited one, referring exclusively to the presence or absence of the patient's capacity to identify himself *fully* with the external reality represented by the patient-therapist relationship" (p. 182, italics by Calef and Weinshel). But again, Calef and Weinshel (1979) indicate how a moment later, Kernberg (1975) claims that "this formulation implies that there is *no continuum,* no gradual shift from presence to absence of reality testing" (p. 182, italics Calef and Weinshel). Calef and Weinshel (1979) conclude:

> If Kernberg accepted some sort of "continuum" between what he describes as the borderline personality and the neurotic, he could point to a series of quantitative and qualitative variations in reality-testing functioning of such patients using the general formulation that with increased regression and deterioration in overall ego integrity there would be a comparable decline in the efficiency of the reality-testing activities. However, since Kernberg holds fast to the idea that this borderline personality organization is a stable and specific psychological entity, he also wants to hold fast to the idea of more specific and more absolute distinctions in the reality-testing functions. (pp. 483-484)

Segal (1981), in what is overall a quite positive evaluation of Kernberg's (e.g., 1975a, 1976) work, fastens on this persistent question of how to formulate some presumably specific type of borderline reality testing from another angle. This has to do with how Kernberg (1975a) uses a concept of splitting. Kernberg contrasts splitting with repression (together with defenses which involve repression) to argue his case that there is something qualitatively different about borderline personality organization in general as well as the reality testing of such individuals in particular. While Kernberg (e.g., 1975a) frequently cites Freud as a source for this concept of splitting, it is Segel's (1981) contention that Freud actually was "describing. . .'disavowal,' not splitting, and that it was only the *effect* of disavowal on the ego that he referred to as a splitting of the ego" (p. 232). Segel (1981) then goes on to make the important point that with this concept of disavowal, Freud always had in mind that reality testing in some way became pathologically altered, whereas in "the splitting as cited by Kernberg, neither of the alternating or antagonistic states of the patient's *need to represent reality*" (p. 232, italics mine).

Segel (1981) raises yet another important consideration about this concept of splitting when he cites some comments made by Freud (1940a) in the Outline:

> The childish ego under the domination of the real world, gets rid of undesireable instinctual demands by what are called repressions. We will now supplement this by further asserting that, during *the same period of life* the ego often

> enough finds itself in the position of fending off some demand from the external world which it feels distressing and that this is effected by means of a disavowal of perceptions which bring to knowledge this demand from reality. Disavowals of this kind occur often enough and not only with fetishists. . . . (pp. 203-204, italics by Segel).

Now Kernberg (e.g., 1975a) certainly conceives of splitting as referring to something which is a qualitatively different process compared to repression, not simply something which is different in terms of external or internal location of psychic danger. Also, splitting for Kernberg (e.g., 1975a) refers to something which belongs decidedly to an earlier developmental context than is true for repression. It is, according to Kernberg (1975a), especially this use of splitting which accounts for the qualitatively different phenomenon which is borderline personality organization. Clearly, then, something must be done here to clarify what at least appears to be an important difference between Freud's (1940a) and Kernberg's (e.g., 1975a) use of this concept of splitting.

It is a thesis of this investigation that both Kernberg and his critics are correct. The critics are correct because I believe it is true that Kernberg has not adequately conceptualized a qualitatively different type of borderline reality testing which is neither like that of a neurotic nor a schizophrenic individual. Without such a conceptualization, Kernberg's contention that there exists a kind of specific and stable personality organization which can be termed "borderline" will not be able to find a secure theoretical basis. I believe it is also true that Kernberg has not attended to the close relationship between these concepts of denial (disavowal) and splitting to be found in Freud's writing; and, consequently, Kernberg does not emphasize enough how a pathological construction of reality must always be involved in any behavior or experience referred to this concept of splitting. Finally, Kernberg really has not provided us with a thorough examination of Freud's writing on the concept of splitting, such that processes of splitting and repression can be conceptualized as separate and different, and as processes which do belong to entirely different developmental contexts.

But Kernberg is correct because I believe he has identified what is really a discrete type of borderline personality organization, and has pointed to the fact that such individuals do manifest a special sort of reality testing disturbance which is neither like that of a neurotic nor a schizophrenic individual. In this investigation I come to define this special sort of borderline reality testing disturbance as a *meaning disturbance.* I can also describe how such a meaning disturbance is, in effect, a kind of "pathological play." By analogy, this can be described as a "perversion" of reality, analogous to perverse corruption of libidinal gratification. The path to this perspective about borderline phenomena is by way of a detailed examination of our psychoanalytic literature about the concepts of splitting and denial (disavowal). But it is a path which also is made possible by Piaget's (e.g., 1945) important research in cognitive development.

This work is also about narcissistic psychopathology. I believe that this same meaning disturbance, especially with respect to how it enables gratifying, playful "illusions" about the reality of self and other, is operative in individuals who are described by Kohut (e.g., 1971, 1977) to exhibit a narcissistic personality disorder. The fact that Kohut (e.g., 1971, 1977) like Kernberg (e.g., 1975a, 1976), places such a great emphasis upon this concept of splitting should at least strongly suggest to us that there may be something essentially similar in both borderline and narcissistic personality disorders.

Also, in this introduction, a word about the organization of this material will be useful. In order to get a "running start" on these issues, I must lay out a place for the concept of splitting within what I consider to be the essentials of a Freudian, psychoanalytic theory of development. This I do in Chapter II. Chapter III then carries over this initial, broad examination into a more detailed study of Piaget's theory of intellectual development as this will later bear upon these concepts of splitting and denial (disavowal).

Chapter IV then takes up and uses the previous material to develop the concept of a meaning disturbance as pathological play. This idea of a meaning disturbance comprehends our familiar concepts of splitting and denial (disavowal) and is seen always to involve psychopathology in reality appraisal. Inasmuch as a meaning disturbance does involve psychopathology in reality appraisal, it is not a neurotic phenomenon. But a meaning disturbance does not involve schizophrenic reconstruction of reality (hallucination or delusion). A meaning disturbance thus involves psychopathology in reality appraisal (relations) which is neither neurotic nor schizophrenic.

Chapter V, in turn, makes use of this concept of a meaning disturbance to describe a comparative psychopathology context for borderline and narcissistic psychopathology. This is to say that at this point I can articulate a place for splitting and denial (disavowal) such that borderline and narcissistic psychopathology can be related to, but also distinguished from, other major types of psychopathology.

The work up to this point has led to a general realization that there exist clinically important variations as to how an individual comes to differentiate and integrate real versus not-real experience. An individual's love, as well as hatred of the loved object, is importantly affected by this matter of real versus not-real meaning, and this topic is taken up in Chapter VI. Chapter VII involves a still further examination of this matter of the different ways in which an individual may come to utilize real or not-real meaning in his or her life. This leads to a concept of *paradoxical creation*. This idea of paradoxical creation can be seen to be relevant to special sorts of conceptual inventiveness (representation) through which an individual (or group) strives to give an eternal meaning to existence, which is, in fact, finite.

Chapter VIII, the last chapter, states summarizing conclusions as well as a comment for clinical practice related to the cognitive perspective emphasized in this investigation.

Three final notes, one about this book's content and the others about its format. This is a book about how certain cognitive considerations which pertain to thinking—representation—affect and are affected by the deep subject matter of psychoanalysis. It is with this perspective that I come to a formulation about splitting and denial, as well as certain other matters which spin off from this formulation. But intelligence, of course, is operative before we acquire a representational capability (Piaget 1936). I have no doubt that for some individuals, what later becomes splitting and denial psychopathology, as I use these terms in connection with representation, already is significantly determined by pathological misuse of intelligence prior to the emergence of representation (see, for example, Freedman, 1980). But I am not aware of any observation such that we must always suppose this to be the case. In any event, this issue is not a topic of this book although I certainly appreciate its importance.

It already will have been noticed that I use the term "denial" (e.g., splitting and denial) and place the term "disavowal" in parentheses (if the latter term appears at all). I am aware that the editors of the *Standard Edition* recommend the English word "disavowal" for the German *verleugnen*. They do this because the English "denial" certainly includes the connotation of a process of negation, which "denial" psychoanalytically is not, and Freud (1925j) used the German *verneinen* in his paper "Negation." But the English "disavowal" includes a connotation which touches upon logical, intellectual (proof and disproof) processes which seem to me to be still further removed from the kind of activity we understand denial to be psychoanalytically. Also, the term "denial" seems to me to admit more easily into expression something which is its opposite, but equally pathological, and this I have come to call "pathological play" (or "playful illusion").

Finally, I have what one might call a footnote fetish. Consequently, footnotes accumulate at a rapid rate. In order to facilitate textual reading, all these footnotes have been collected, placed at the end of the text, and are organized there by chapter.

2

On Splitting and the Psychoanalytic Concept of Development

I want, at the beginning, to establish some boundaries. My immediate aim is to examine the relationship between the idea of splitting and a psychoanalytic conception of development. I want, so to speak, to locate this idea of splitting among certain major concepts which constitute certain essentials of a psychoanalytic theory of development. When I speak of development, I have in mind both its occurrence and its nonoccurrence, and the nonoccurrence of development represents the most general statement we can make about psychopathology. I will take up in this chapter the following conceptual matters, roughly in this order: (1) The idea of development itself, and related to this, concepts of differentiation, integration, and emergence. (2) The relationship between self theory, especially espoused by Kohut (e.g., 1971, 1977), and psychic system theory (e.g., Freud, 1923b). Or, better stated, I will address the controversy about this matter in recent literature (e.g., Ornstein, 1974) and take a position myself which I believe leaves us with a more effective, psychoanalytic conception of development. (3) Finally, I will take up some of Freud's (1920g) most basic ideas about development: the pleasure and reality principles, the life and death instincts, as well as the repetition compulsion. After all of this, I will suggest a location for the idea of splitting within a psychoanalytic conception of development. But what first will be useful are some introductory comments about this concept of splitting.

Has psychoanalytic theory gotten "high" on the concept of splitting? Pruyser (1975), in a review of the literature, answers this question with a resounding "Yes." Splitting, Pruyser tells us, is both a "tricky" (p. 43) and a "slippery" (p. 44) word: It lulls our critical sense and promotes an illusion that we understand. Pruyser contends that a good hard look at this concept of splitting reveals it to be "extremely indefinite" (p. 44) in terms of what it is supposed to mean. I agree with Pruyser that this concept of splitting extends in our literature like some lush, overgrown, jungle vine. It becomes increasingly difficult to disentangle the many meanings of the term. Lustmann (1977), in a still more recent review, concludes that the literature on splitting involves "multiple, partial, and parallel theoretical models of underlying process—all separated by profound, unexamined differences in conceptual vocabulary and tradition[11] (p. 124). Moreover, I believe meanings have become attached to the idea of splitting which are inherently contradictory. Further, if we use this idea of splitting to describe what is considered to be a typical, natural way of thinking in the young child, then I think we bear witness to a false extrapolation from psychopathology to normal development. It was Winnicott (1953) who realized that the earliest mental constructions of the young child must, in a certain way, first be accepted and go unchallenged. Then a child will progress naturally into an ultimate objectification of experience which will be felt by the child as his or her own construction (not imposed). Perhaps there is something special about this concept of splitting, or psychoanalytic theory altogether, that requires (by analogy) a similar "developmental line" (A. Freud, 1965, p. 64). I think that Pruyser's (1975) criticism does signal a timely effort to refine a concept which has, indeed, grown rampant in our literature. But I consider that Pruyser's final injunction that the concept of splitting should be "banned" (p. 44) is to throw the baby out with the bath water.

On the other hand, the position about splitting that I will develop in this investigation also will not be consistent with that of Lustmann (1977). Lustmann not only favors retention of this concept but employs it in varying contexts of normal development, and thus clinical health, as well as in different sorts of psychopathology. I will argue for a conception of splitting which always implicates psychopathology. At the same time, I will come to understand this concept of splitting in a way which I believe promotes a more general, theoretical comprehension about *vicissitudes of real and not-real construction.* In fact, I believe that it is because the concept of splitting can be exploited for such theoretical purpose that Freud (e.g., 1894a, 1923e, 1925j, 1927e, 1933a, 1940a) constantly was drawn back to this idea. Thus, I believe this idea of splitting does describe something real and important which only psychoanalysis could have learned through its study of adult psychopathology and normal as well as abnormal child development. But an infatuation with this idea of splitting in our literature has made very fuzzy, indeed, the nature of this important reality.

I take it for granted that splitting, as would be true for any kind of psychopathology, involves the contribution of instinctual drive conflicts as well as determinants which have to do with matters pertinent to object relationships, and that, as well, narcissistic dynamics contribute to the occurrence of splitting. However, my interest now is not with the *clinical etiology* of splitting. My attempt here is only to understand, theoretically, what sort of meaning the idea of splitting can possess from the perspective of a psychoanalytic conception of development. But also, I want to understand what kind of psychoanalytic theory of development we should possess which will enable us to provide this idea of splitting with a clear and distinct meaning, and a meaning which adds to our overall theoretical realization about the phenomenon of development.

I did not, in my comments about the clinical etiology of splitting, refer to another determinant, and this is the contribution of what Freud (1900a) called the "psychical apparatus" (p. 538). Roughly, but I think adequately for my purposes here, I will say that Freud's (1900a) concept of a "psychical apparatus" (p. 538) corresponds to the totality of those psychic events which produce meaning. I thus will talk about a *meaning-making* or *meaning-producing* apparatus. I do not say that meaning production is more or less critical as a determinant for the clinical etiology of splitting as compared to those other factors I already have described. But I do say that splitting, as a particular kind of psychopathology, especially and uniquely shows itself as a disturbance in meaning production. If splitting means anything, it means something about whether there occurs an expected structuralization with regard to a core area of self (and object) *representation* which pertains to matters of emotional esteem, survival, and the like. I am talking about something which Freud (1900a) also once described simply as "thought structures" (p. 542). Hartmann (1939), over forty years ago, emphasized how the origin and development of such a meaning-making apparatus cannot be said to be derived from "relationships of instinctual drives or love objects, but are rather *prerequisites* of our conception of these and their development" (p. 15). Hartmann (1939) spoke about "learning to think" (p. 14). And it was, of course, Hartmann (1939) who emphasized how thinking must be understood as one of a number of "independent biological functions which exist alongside, and *in part* independent of, instinctual drives" (p. 14, italics mine).

But Hartmann's perfectly clear theoretical statement about the existence of such codeterminants of behavior and experience, each of which undergoes a quasi-autonomous development, has only, with a few useful exceptions (e.g.,Anthony, 1956; Bion, 1954; Fraiberg, 1969; Gould, 1972; Grubbs, 1981; Schachtel, 1947; Schimek, 1975; Schmid-Kitsikis, 1976; Steingart, 1969; Wolf, 1967), been given a kind of lip service in our literature. It is certainly useful, for example, to acknowledge that a necessary but insufficient condition for superego system formation is an advance in thinking from "concretistic object and self imagery to that [which is] more conceptual." (Jacobson, 1964, p. 126). But this kind of formulation stops right at the point in which any detailed investigation would begin; this is how it is that changes in "learning to think" (Hartmann, 1939, p. 14) codetermine the structuralization of self and object representations into the psychic system superego. What is critical here is how this "concretistic imagery" is *organized.* Concepts infiltrated with "concretistic imagery" may or may not be indicative of immature thought (e.g., Kris, 1952).

It is now time for a definition. The following definition by Kernberg (1975a) supports my emphasis that splitting is pathological meaning production in self (and object) representation, and is consistent with current literature (e.g., Mahler, 1968; Kohut, 1971; Lichtenberg and Slap, 1973).

> Introjections and identifications established under the influence of libidinal drive derivatives are at first built up separately from those established under the influence of aggressive drive derivatives ("good" and "bad" internal ob-

> jects, or "positive" and "negative" introjections). This division . . . happens at first simply because of the lack of integrative capacity of the early ego. Later on, what originally was a lack of integrative capacity is used defensively by the emerging ego in order to prevent the generalization of anxiety . . . *A simple defect in integration is then used actively for other purposes.* . . . This mechanism is normally used only in an early stage of ego development during the first year of life, and rapidly is replaced by higher level defensive operations of the ego which center around repression. . . . (p.25)
>
> In contrast, in pathological conditions this mechanism [splitting] persists. . . . The drive derivative . . . attains full emotional, ideational, and motor consciousness, but is completely separated from other segments of the conscious psychic experience. Under these pathological circumstances, contradictory ego states are alternatively activated [and] anxiety is prevented. (pp. 25-26)

I agree with such a description of splitting as far as it goes, in terms of the meaning production which is splitting. But notice that there is nothing in this definition which emphasizes the pertinence of splitting to the maintenance of belief which is in some way not-real; this point, recently stressed by Segel (1980), and earlier by Stewart (1970), is something to which I will return later in this investigation. Now, I want to criticize certain implications about development which also inhere in this description of splitting.

In the first place, to say that a young child who conceptualizes experience on the basis of vivid qualities of "good" versus "bad," pleasure versus pain, or what not, shows a lack of integration, is adultomorphic. Actually, thinking, even such global concepts as "good," "bad," or what not is a momentous integrative achievement which *emerges* out of exclusively sensorimotor intelligence (Piaget, 1936). Such concepts as "good," "bad," and so forth can be described as a normal and natural differentiation process with respect to development yet to be accomplished, and integration with respect to development already accomplished. This is not to play around with words, but a necessary way of stating things when one uses a theory of development which works with ideas of differentiation and integration that produce progressively more complex and *emergent* psychic organization (function and content). The development of meaning structures is no different in this regard from the ontogeny of any skill in the life cycle, say, motor skills. A substantive point here is that processes of differentation and integration characterize all stages of human development. Indeed, for psychoanalysis, *the idea of development itself* is inconceivable without some such notions about differentiating and integrating processes which produce successively more complex, emergent, psychic structure (function and content). A related substantive point is that these processes of differentiation and integration, in themselves, undergo emergent change with development, something very much appreciated by Hartmann (1947). It was Hartmann (1947) who suggested, for example, that Nunberg's (1930) concept of a synthetic (integrative) function be understood to apply only when an individual's experience and behavior have reached an order of complexity such that we conceptualize a psychic system ego as an ordering abstraction.

I return to Kernberg's (1975a) description of splitting as something initially due to "a lack of integration," which later is used "actively" to "prevent anxiety" (p. 25). I believe that to regard splitting as a clinically normal mental activity in early childhood condenses, in a not-fruitful way, the idea of early natural kinds of differentiation and integration processes with something that is better always left for a depiction of defense and psychopathology.

It is another thing for a young child to conceptualize experience into that which means pleasure versus that which means pain, or "good" versus "bad," or whatever, because the only procedures for meaning organization available to the child make such classification a natural outcome. For example, Freud (1915c) once hypothesized the emergence of a stage in mental constructions such that oneself means everything pleasureable—Freud (1915c) called this a "pleasure-ego" (p. 136)—and psychic pain means not-self. My point is that I believe that here Freud believed he was describing a natural, clinically healthy and normal development in meaning organization. I believe this is the reason that Freud never once used the idea of splitting in his description of such mental constructions although the term "splitting" had already been part of his published, theoretical vocabulary for over twenty years (Freud 1894a).

I return once more to Kernberg's (1975a) description of splitting, and this time my attention is upon his use of the psychic system term "ego" in connection with splitting: "This mechanism . . . [i.e., splitting] . . . is normally used only in an early stage of ego development during the first year of life" (p. 25). Freud (1914c) stated: "The unity comparable to the ego cannot exist in the individual from the start; the ego has to be developed" (p. 77). And Freud (1926c) also stated: "The ego is an organization. It is based on the maintenance . . . of reciprocal influence between all its parts" (p. 98). So, what immediately rises in one's mind is whether it is theoretically appropriate to use this psychic system term "ego," even with the qualification "early stage of ego development," in connection with the concept of splitting.

We are accustomed, indeed required because of certain psychoanalytic observations about neurotic experience and behavior, to conceptualize certain processes of differentiation and integration which result in id, ego, and superego psychic systems (structures). But processes of differentiation and integration characterize all stages of human development. As I already have stated, the idea of development itself is inconceivable without some such notions about differentiating and integrating processes, and it is exactly this which distinguishes living development in nature from inanimate matter (e.g., Murphy, 1947). It is easy enough to document in our literature how such an orientation characterizes our *entire* psychoanalytic theory of development. This includes earlier periods of the life cycle which eventuate into id, ego, and superego, the "centers of psychic functioning" (Hartmann, Kris, and Lowenstein, 1947, p. 14), as well as continued personality development subsequent to the emergence of these psychic systems.

For example, Jacobson (1964) asks us to conceive of an "initial. . .undifferentiated psychophysical energy . . . [which differentiates into] . . . the libidinal and aggressive drives with which the id is endowed" (p. 14). Schur (1966) considers such an idea congruent with a more general conception that the id as a psychic structure emerges out of development and is subject to subsequent development. Freud (1915e) explicitly stated that the dynamic unconscious is "capable of development" (p. 191). And Freud (1915d) also recognized how, once developed as a psychic system, the id will continue to develop through integration because "repression does not hinder the instinctual representative from continuing to exist in the unconscious, from *organizing itself* further, putting out derivatives and establishing connections" (p. 149, italics mine). Holt (1967) has provided another example of how Freud regarded a type of integrative activity to be present in the id, and this has to do with Freud's (1912x) description of animistic thinking as a *system* of thought (p.77, italics mine). More particularly, Freud's (1915d) recognition that a kind of integrative activity is evident in primary-process thinking is shown in his description of displacement as something which takes place "along the chain of associations which is *determined in a particular way*" (p. 155, italics mine).

With regard to the psychic system ego, Freud understood that reality testing, which eventually becomes an ego system function, is not achieved "all at once" (1911b, p. 222), and that it is a product of differentiation. Freud also pointed to integrative activities as sources for the psychic system ego. He described, for example, how what ultimately becomes the ego system's function of defense against an instinctually internal demand "will be modeled on the defense adopted against an *external* stimulus" (Freud, 1926d, p. 92). Hartmann's (1939) concept of "secondary autonomy" (p. 26) is one idea among others (e.g., Erikson 1950) which theoretically documents how the psychic system ego continues to develop subsequent to its initial emergence.

With regard to what becomes the superego system function of raising moral and ideal demands (Hartmann and Lowenstein, 1962), we understand how early differentiating and integrating processes can contribute to the achievement of this psychic system. For example, Jacobson (1964) points to the necessity for the young child first to be able to differentiate between wished-for versus actual self representations. Early integrative activities which produce an eventual superego psychic system also are illustrated by Jacobson (1964) when she describes the young child's process of "blending" (p. 92) of all representations which relate to goal setting and aspirations. Once established, we understand theoretically how the system superego normally continues to develop, to become "more imper sonal" (Freud, 1933a, p. 295), and also how it is capable of relatively autonomous function (Hartmann and Lowenstein, 1962). Novey (1955b), as well as Loewald (1962a), conceptualizes the system superego as an enduring psychic structure which normally includes continuous movement of mental content which is experienced as fully realized into the psychic system ego; there is, then, a kind of continuous replacement of goal setting and ideal content into the superego system.

These comments only signal another, larger, and presently hotly argued question about what a proper psychoanalytic conception of development is. This is the question of self theory versus psychic system theory. Gedo and Goldberg (1973) recently have argued that *none* of our psychic system terms are an appropriate framework for pre-Oedipal experience and behavior, and with this I agree. In fact, what is occurring in our literature as a conceptual framework for this earlier period of life has to do with attributes of self and object representation (e.g., Kernberg, 1975a; Mahler, 1968; Mahler, Pine, and Bergman, 1975; Lichenstein, 1964; Kohut, 1971, 1977; Levin, 1969). However, while our psychic system conceptualization is not an adequate framework for early childhood, I believe that our theoretical conceptualization about self and object representation applies throughout the life cycle, although in different ways in early versus later childhood and adulthood. I now want to explicate a viewpoint about the relationship between self construct theory and our psychic system terminology.

A substantive point is this: It is the task of a developmental psychoanalytic psychology to document theoretically both *emergent change and continuity* in the life cycle, and it must accomplish this for *both psychic content and psychic function.* Certainly, the very data produced by the practice of psychoanalysis—the uncovering of genetic determinants, historical reconstruction, character analysis, and so forth—force the theory of psychoanalysis to account for both historical continuity in the life cycle and emergent change. The commitment of psychoanalysis, as a developmental psychology, to such a conjoint historical-continuity-emergent viewpoint, is already perfectly clear in Freud's (1905d) early theory of psychosexual development. Psychosexual development involves, of course, the idea of emergent stages. The concept of forepleasure has to do with a transformed, i.e., emergent, use and content for infantile sexuality in genital sexuality (endpleasure). But, at the same time, how an adult (mis)uses infantile forepleasure in his or her genital sexuality always will reveal something about his or her psychosexual history.[1]

I already have suggested elsewhere (Steingart, 1969) a way to begin to integrate our constructs about self and object representation with our psychic system theory. We can understand our id, ego, and superego systems to be concepts which signal an emergent differentiation of psychic function. But such an emergent differentiation is inconceivable without an accompanying idea of emergent integration of psychic function, and this is nothing else but the concept of character (see, for example, Fenichel, 1945). I conceive of character to implicate the existence of our most complex integrative psychic organization (Steingart, 1969), and such an integrative structure pertains to the psychic systems which "are not conceived of as independent parts of personality . . . but as three centers of psychic functioning" (Hartmann, Kris, and Lowenstein, 1947, p. 14).

For example, observation certainly leads us to conclude that a good deal of the time a little, clinically healthy child vigorously is attempting to fulfill some wished-for representation of him or herself, and/or attempting in some way to obtain parental approval (or avoidance of disapproval), and that all together such efforts can raise the child's self-esteem. We consider that this entire endeavor to fulfill wishful ideals, and/or parental approval, becomes with development a more or less coherent psychic organization itself, and we term this a superego. If we want, psychoanalytically, we can reserve the term values or value formation as something which only applies to such an emergent differentiation of psychic function. But values, now regarded as a sign for the emergence of the psychic system superego, also must be considered to be integrated throughout an entire personality. For example, we expect our values to influence our adaptation to reality, i.e., the manner in which we perceive, think, etc. Statements similar to what I have just said could be written about the developmental acquisition of the psychic systems ego and id.

But character must possess an integrative achievement for the content of self representation as well. Self representation content cannot only be ascribed to the separate, differentiated psychic systems; but there exists, as well, a self representation content for this integrative formation of psychic function, which is character itself. I also already have suggested (Steingart, 1969) that it would clarify matters to restrict our concept of *the* self to this acquisition of integrative content for self representation, which goes together with integrated psychic function as character, i.e., that we consider *the* self to be a late latency phenomenon which follows upon early childhood Oedipal resolution. I believe that Hartmann's (1953) comment about the "self-image . . . (a *complex* of representations)" (italics mine, p. 192) implies this kind of concept about such an emergent, integrative phenomenon in self representation content.

Specifically then, with respect to our construct of *the* self, we describe something about the integrative organization of a whole personality in terms of self representation content; whereas when we describe something in terms of integrative psychic function, we talk about character. To be sure, some content of the self representation is accessible to consciousness, while other content will be located in the dynamic unconscious. But the fact that there is self representation content in the dynamic unconscious does not *necessarily* lead to a conclusion that an integration of *the* self has not been achieved. With our concept of sublimation, for example, we obviously describe what we consider to be a positive state of affairs in which what remains dynamically unconscious mental content is adaptively integrated into the representation of *the* self. But even with respect to psychopathology, we ought to emphasize more than we do that our concept of conflict is not identical with our concept of integration (Steingart, 1969). Certainly, dynamically unconscious mental content pertinent to the representation of the self is involved in conflictual experience and/or behavior. But if we clinically identify such conflict to be neurotic, then we believe that there exist the essentials of differentiation and integration with regard to mature personality organization. Indeed, in such a circumstance we can and should say that conflict itself has undergone an emergent transformation. We indicate this *systemic* framework for conflict with concepts like "intra-psychic conflict" (e.g., Moore and Fine, 1968) or "intersystemic conflict" (e.g., Hartmann, 1950, p. 138), and we say that this will register for an individual as experience or behavior which is felt as *ego*-alien (e.g., Fenichel, 1945, p. 453, italics mine); that is, not simply psychicly painful but something which is experienced in a special way as a violation of systemic activity.

In other words, if we now only consider a post-Oedipal, late latency period of personality, our concepts of id, ego, and superego are not more abstract, less experiential, or whatever, compared with our constructs of *the* self; and *the* self is not a separate and special agency or viewpoint compared to our psychic systems (see, for example, Levin, 1969; Lichtenberg, 1975; Lustmann, 1977; Kohut, 1971, 1977; Abend, 1974). Altogether then, my comments about self representation sum up to the following conclusions with respect to a coordination between my proposed use of the self construct and our psychic system (id, ego, superego) terminology: We deal here with a matter of the psychic reality of differentiated psychic structures as well as the psychic reality of their integration, together with a matter of whether our description is about the psychic function or content.[2] I also now suggest that we adopt and use Erikson's (1950) term "identity" (p. 227) to apply only to that special awareness about change and continuity in the content of the self which characterizes adolescence. This, I believe, highlights the essence of what Erikson (e.g., 1950) intended in his introduction of the term identity (see also Blos, e.g., 1977).

On the other hand, if we consider only the pre-Oedipal period, we have constructs about the attributes of self (and object) representation which carry for us not only ideas about psychic content, but also ideas about psychic function in early childhood. But to contrast or raise an issue about psychic system theory *versus* self-construct terminology, with respect to early childhood, is not even to compare apples with pears. It is to compare apples with nothing. The substantive point here is this: The experience and behavior of the young child has not yet developed to a point of (inferred) psychic structural complexity such that certain emergent psychic function(s) (e.g., self-criticism) and psychic content(s) (e.g., guilt) occur which require psychic system terms as ordering abstractions. If we did not have our id, ego, and superego psychic systems concepts, we would have to invent some other terms to perform this theoretical task for us in order to deal with the kind of psychic structural complexity which emerges with development.

To return again to the post-Oedipal, late latency child and adult, some (e.g., Kohut, 1977; Lustmann, 1978) have said that to infer a self construct from psychic content is to mark it as closer to immediate experience than a psychic system term like ego. This has to do with a confusion between what is meant by immediate experience and what is meant by psychic content in psychoanalysis. In actuality, the psychic content of psychoanalysis does not mean the immediate personal experience of the analysand, which is, hopefully, empathically reproduced in the analyst. Psychic content is a *construction* made from such immediate experience—that the experience *means* anger, love, sexual excitement, etc., which already is a different thing. Psychic content is experience *which can be communicated because it possesses meaning.* Meaning requires activities performed by the psychic apparatus, such as remembering, concentration, etc., which support another critical activity—some kind of conceptualization—which provides such meaning.

It is, of course, Kohut (1971) who has been led from an initial consideration that narcissism "follows an independent line" (p. 6) to a further conclusion that a "new. . .psychology of the self" (Kohut 1977, p. 22) is required. According to Kohut (1977), there is needed a new psychology of the self which goes beyond the psychology "of the self in the narrow sense, in which the self is seen as a content of a mental apparatus" (p. xvi). One gathers from such a statement that it is "narrow" to view conceptualization about self representation only as mental content, and indeed Kohut (1977) means this clearly in comments I will cite injust a moment. But first I want to emphasize that the mental contents of self representation are anything but "narrow" with respect to the various systems of psychic function, and I only repeat here something already made clear by Hartmann (1950):

> We actually do find "narcissism" in all three psychic systems. . . . It therefore will be clarifying if we define narcissism as the libidinal cathexis not of the ego but of the self. (It might also be useful to apply the term of self representation as opposed to object representation.) (p. 127)

In other words, self representation and narcissism, which is a positive libidinal cathexsis of such mental content, are a matter which has pertinence to an individual's *total* psychic functioning.

Now the citation from Kohut (1977):

> The framework of the structural model of the mind, even when employed in conjunction with the most sophisticated ego-psychological elaborations of drive psychology, is not sufficiently pertinent . . . [and] we must introduce a new framework . . . [for] the psychology of the self—a psychology that deals

> with the formation *and functions of the self,* and with its break-up and reintegration. (p. 22, italics mine)

It is easy enough to see that Kohut (1977) here maintains that a self theory must be accepted which has to do not simply with mental content but psychic function as well, i.e., "functions of the self" (Kohut, 1977, p. 22); and that our terminology about id, ego, and superego structures of psychic function cannot suffice.

I believe this "separatist" position of Kohut's (1977) could be justified if one were to portray the relationship between mental apparatus psychic function and psychic content as being like the relationship between a movie projector and a film strip. Here, the apparatus of the movie projector stands for the mental apparatus which enables a variety of psychic functions which we conceptualize according to id, ego, and superego systems. The film strip is the equivalent of self representation mental content, and we need a proper operation of the projector to obtain film strip content. But the substantive point here is that there is no *indigenous* relationship between the movie projector apparatus which enables psychic functions and the self representation contents of the film strip. *The movie projector does not create the film strip content out of properties which inhere in its own functioning.* If one of Skinner's (1951) fabulous pigeons that were trained to play ping-pong were strong enough, swift enough, and could be taught to pull a film strip at the right rate of speed, at the right angle, past a hand-held lens, etc., then we also could obtain our film strip content. A better model, indeed one closer to the reality of human beings, is that of a computer as a psychic apparatus which enables psychic functions and its *production* of information as self representation content. Here there is an indigenous relationship between apparatus function and content. Information is produced by the computer out of properties intrinsic to its own functional capabilities. Extraordinarily miniaturized circuits, implanted on chips, may or may not be activated by electron switches; such on–off circuitry can enable a representation of the numbers one or zero, and out of these basic representations more complex information can be constructed. Certainly we can and must have information terminology, as well as conceptualization which has to do with the computer apparatus functioning, but all of these attributes are ingredients of this same computer.

Consider another mechanical illustration: Let us say that we have before us both a color and a black-and-white television set. The color television set literally provides us not just with more information, but with an entirely different order of mental content, i.e., color in contrast to black and white. We can say that the qualitatively different information provided by the color television set corresponds to the higher order of mental content possessed by a human adult, whereas the black-and-white picture corresponds to the more limited mental content possessed, say, by an adult ape. But it is clear that in both cases the different orders of mental content—black-and-white versus color information—are provided by, that is, are indigenous and organic to certain characteristics of each television set apparatus. In the case of the color television set, there exist apparatuses for a differentiation and integration of the three primary colors, whereas the black-and-white set does not possess such apparatuses. I believe all of what I have just said is consistent with Freud's view, and that this is why he used the same term, ego, to refer to both psychic function and, implicitly, mental content.

I am not altogether happy with these mechanical similes, and I want to make clear that I do not intend by them any examination of the mind-body problem. I am describing psychological matters: A human being is born with a species-specific potential for a development of certain motor, perceptual, thinking, etc., capabilities—what Hartmann (1939) called "mental apparatuses" (p. 100). Altogether, these apparatuses are what Freud (1900a) meant by the "psychical apparatus" (p. 540); in part, they determine and are determined by drive, narcissistic, and object relationship factors (Hartmann, 1939). A species-specific, human ontogenesis of psychic structure is the result of all of these determinants which enter into development. These psychic structures become evident to us by the performance of psychic function and the production of psychic content which is indigenous to such mental apparatus psychic functioning. A mental apparatus of the human being is what I have termed a meaning apparatus. Some kind of self and object representation content will occur which is indigenous to the way only a human can produce meaning. And a psychic function which only a human *may* come to perform, for example, self-criticism, also is indigenous to such a psychic apparatus. No other animal can produce self and object representation content and function about self-criticism in the way a human can.

But no general, theoretical comments about the idea of development can be complete without consideration of what Freud (1911b) called "principles of mental function" (p. 218). What I must do now is compare and contrast Freud's (1911b) initial set of concepts about basic principles of mental function, pleasure and reality principles, with his later formulated (Freud, 1920g) ideas about the life and death instinct.

To begin with the pleasure principle (Freud, 1911b), it is clear enough what Freud meant by this. It is also clear how the reality principle, at this point, represents no fundamental departure from this idea of mental function as involving a psychic apparatus which operates to bring about discharge, with an attendant conscious experience of gratification.

> I . . . suggest that the state of psychical rest, i.e., no tension, was originally disturbed by the pre-emptory demands of internal needs. Whenever this happened, whatever was thought of (wished for) was simply presented in hallucinatory manner. . . . It was only the non-occurrence of the expected satisfaction. . . that led to the abandonment of this attempt. . . . Instead of it, the psychical apparatus had to decide to form a conception of the real circumstances . . . and to endeavor to make a real alteration in them. A new principle

> of mental functioning was thus introduced . . . the *reality principle* . . . (p. 219)
>
> Actually, the substitution of the reality principle for the pleasure principle implies no deposing of the pleasure principle but only a safeguarding of it. A momentary pleasure, uncertain in its results, is given up but only in order to gain. . .an assured pleasure at a later time. (p. 223)

Of course, Freud (1911b) realized that "a slave to the [tension reduction] pleasure principle . . . could not maintain itself alive for the shortest time" (p. 220). He himself responded to this point by saying that "a fiction like this is however justified . . . provided one includes with it the care it [the infant] receives from its mother." (Freud, 1911b, p. 220) Freud then went on to liken the human infant state, in a famous metaphor, to the situation of the unborn chick within the maternal egg. However, the operative question here is not physical survival but psychic *development*. Clearly, what it is that develops is some type of anticipatory *capability:* "A momentary pleasure . . . is given up to gain an assured pleasure *at a later time*" (Freud, 1911b, p. 223, italics mine). What makes this critical is that this is an account of the acquisition of a *relationship*, that is, between "momentary pleasure" and pleasure at "a later time." Hartmann (1939) has indicated how nothing in the immediate, subjective qualities of a pleasure or pain experience can produce such a means-end—that is, anticipatory—representation. Or, to put it in Hartmann's (1939) words, there is a "function of anticipating" (p. 43) which must enter as an "independent factor" (p. 44) in psychic development. But while Hartmann (1939) thus argued for the existence of "something essentially new" (p. 43), besides the pleasure principle, as a determinant of mental development, he did not "enthrone" any other principle of mental function equal in significance to the pleasure principle for individual (contrasted to Homo sapiens species) development.

But actually Freud (1920g) had done this himself in his monograph *Beyond the Pleasure Principle*. There is something extraordinarily disconcerting about a reading of *Beyond the Pleasure Principle* (Freud, 1920g). But this is not simply because Freud introduces such a grave idea as the death instinct. It is as if one were watching a titanic shell game played by a grand master with shells involving death as well as life; and yet one's conceptual eye is somehow kept riveted upon the development of the idea of the death instinct. But what really happens which is of such extraordinary importance is that to his usual formulation of the pleasure principle (including its modification known as the reality principle), Freud now adds another entirely different principle of mental function for individual (as well as for Homo sapiens species) development.

I take up here something already suggested by Ricoeur (1970), but especially emphasized by Loewald (1973). Freud's (1920g) well-known development of the idea of a death instinct proceeds in three steps. Freud first identified something which is solid clinical observation—"a compulsion to repeat" (p. 19)—and of course what he emphasized was the repetition in the transference of "past experiences which include no possibility of pleasure, and which can *never* [have] brought satisfaction even to instinctual impulses which have since been repressed" (p. 20, italics mine). Freud next considered that one way to understand this compulsion to repeat would be to see it as an effort to "*master* the stimulus retrospectively, [which was the cause] of the traumatic neurosis" (p. 32, italics mine). Such an effort to master a disturbing stimulus, Freud said, would not operate "in *opposition* to the pleasure principle, but independently of it and to some extent in disregard of it" (p. 35). The straightforward idea here is that such mastery is a kind of pre-condition. Only when such mastery "has been accomplished would it be possible for the dominance of the pleasure principle . . . to proceed unhindered" (p. 35). But now Freud took the final, decisive step and applied the "predicate of being 'instinctual' . . . to the compulsion to repeat" (p. 36). Freud conducted a wide-ranging examination about life and death phenomena throughout evolution. He concluded, in an admittedly speculative fashion, that a "universal attribute of instincts and perhaps of organic life in general is . . . *to restore an earlier state of things*" (p. 36); at another time, Freud (1924c) described this as an aim "to conduct the restlessness of life into the stability of the inorganic state" (p. 160). Thus we have Thanatos, the death instinct. But Loewald (1973) already has pointed out how such a conception of the death instinct fundamentally is *no change at all* from the idea of a tension-reduction principle of mental function. It is only "beyond" the pleasure principle in that Freud carries this idea of tension-reduction to a kind of ultimate conclusion, which is to do away with life inasmuch as tension is inherent in life itself.

What *is different* is a *new* formulation by Freud of the sexual instincts, which he now terms Eros. These sexual instincts, Freud says, are the "true life instincts. They operate against the purposes of . . . death" (Freud, 1920g, p. 40). From now on, in Freud's writing, the relationship between something still called the pleasure (tension-reduction) principle and the libidinal drives really is no longer the same. As Loewald (1973) puts it, this change in viewpoint is, at least in part, due to Freud's finally capitulating before the fact that stimulus tension is, in and of itself, "*not necessarily* unpleasurable and a state which tends to be avoided" (p. 14, italics mine). Nowhere is this clearer than in Freud's comments, written four years later, in his paper "The Economic Problem of Masochism" (1924c):

> It cannot be doubted that there are pleasurable tensions and unpleasurable relaxations of tension. The state of sexual excitement is the most striking example . . . but it is certainly not the only one. (p. 160).
>
> Pleasure and unpleasure, therefore, cannot be referred simply to an increase or decrease of a quantity. . . .It appears that they depend . . . on some characteristic . . . we can only describe as a qualitative one. . . . We do not know. (p. 160)

So we come to a point of recognition that these concepts of a life and death instinct really have to do with radically opposed characteristics of the human organism with regard to psychic tension, one to *use* psychic tension *for development* of psychic structure (and this means psychic function as well as content), the other to avoid and reduce such tension. Any subjective experience of some variety of psychic pleasure or pain is complexly related to these two principles of mental function (Freud, 1924c; see also Jacobson [1953a] for a more recent, cogent emphasis about this matter). Anna Freud (1960) has stated about the pleasure principle, now understood as a principle of tension-reduction in mental function, that "as such *it is not a drive representation at all* . . . in its metapsychological sense it is conceived as a principle which governs *all* mental activity" (p. 55, italics mine). I believe the same reasoning must apply to the radically new principle of mental function which Freud (1929g) introduced with the term "life instinct." That is, the so-called life instinct also is not a drive representation at all but another basic principle of mental function which also applies to all mental activity.

From Freud's (1920g) changed, and now genuinely dual, principles of mental function, there follows a changed conception about how we acquire representation (thought). There is a generalization to be drawn from Hartmann's (1939) contention that anticipation enters as an "independent factor" (p. 44), and cannot be understood to inhere in something about the qualities of pleasure or pain, which then is automatically to be referred to a conceptualization that there is a rise or fall in psychic tension. This generalization is that representation (a concept)—however immature or mature, and whether it be real or not real—presupposes a consciousness which possesses knowledge about the existence of a fundamental category of *similarity* (Cassirer, 1953; Wallach, 1958; Nelson, 1974). Knowledge about such similarity is a construction which provides meaning and does not inhere in any of the immediate qualities of psychic pleasure or pain. Similarity knowledge also has to do with a relating function (Hartmann 1939), inasmuch as a particular pleasure or pain experience (or whatever) is *known* to be referrable to another experience on the basis of some identity; and so an *idea* (some type of concept) is acquired.[3] Here we must consider that there operates that other fundamental mental principle (life instinct) which uses psychic tension for the construction of a meaning structure.

A well-known clinical observation related to all of this, and one which I think especially illuminates the significance of the "compulsion to repeat" (Freud, 1920g, p. 19) as it applies to the acquisition of thought, is the so-called "resistance to change" (Wing, 1972, p. 72) of autistic children. This is a phenomenon which, since the very beginning of pertinent clinical observation (Wittmer 1919–22), has marked this diagnosis. To state this matter positively, autistic children characteristically show panicky and/or enraged reactions if some sort of favored activity with an inanimate object, or some preferred physical arrangement, etc., is changed in the slightest degree. While object relations and dynamic psychoanalytic theory certainly can and must be applied to such a phenomenon, any such explanation is incomplete without a consideration which takes into account the acquisition of the fundamental construction of the similarity category for human experience and behavior. I believe that what autistic children demonstrate in their rigid and poignant repetitive effort to maintain tangible, concrete sameness is a fundamental disturbance in their acquisition of a *mental* category of psychological similarity necessary for the emergence of thought (conception).

But this "compulsion to repeat" (Freud, 1920g, p. 19) will obtain even further clarification if we understand it to be not only pertinent to human development. In fact, the "compulsion to repeat" (Freud, 1920g, p. 19) is a phenomenon which signals disturbance in what would be the expected, progressive development of any reasonably complex organism in interaction with its natural milieu. Thomas (1974), for example, describes such repetitive behavior on the part of the solitary wasp Sphex, when what would otherwise be a certain natural progression of egg-laying behavior is interfered with by experimental manipulation:

> The solitary wasp Sphex, nearing her time of eggs, travels aloft with a single theory about caterpillars. Finding one to match the hypothesis, she swoops, pins it, paralyzes it, carries it off, and descends to deposit it precisely in front of the door of the round burrow . . . she had prepared beforehand. . . . She drops the beast, enters the burrow, inspects the interior for last-minute irregularities, then comes out to pull it in for the egg-laying. . . . But if, while she is inside, . . . you move the caterpillar a short distance, she has a less sensible second thought. . . . She emerges, searches for a moment, finds it, drags it back to the original spot, drops it again, and runs inside to check the burrow again. If you move the caterpillar again, she will repeat the program, and you can keep her totally preoccupied for as long as you have the patience and the heart for it. It is a *compulsive, essentially neurotic kind of behavior* . . . (p. 109, italics mine)

The point of my presentation of these observations is hardly to equate repetitious egg-laying behavior with the actions of an autistic child repetitiously struggling, I believe, to achieve a fundamental mental category of similarity. But it is to argue that disturbance in what otherwise would be an expected progression of a reasonably complex organism's development in its natural milieu will show itself in unproductive, repetitious behavior relevant to the organism so involved. Other such examples easily could be cited from the animal kingdom (see, for example, Beer's [1962] work with black-headed gulls). This is not because of any universal tendency among life forms to return to an earlier, inorganic condition, as Freud (1920g) suggested. Rather, reasonably complex organisms, including Homo sapiens, are simply *designed* so as to behave repetitively and unproductively—to sputter—when development which is natural to a species is prevented by pathology. Also, it perhaps does no great harm to apply Freud's (1920g) other idea, an effort to "master" (p. 32), to this circumstance. However, what has to be kept clear is that we are not describing psychoanalytically understood motivation but, rather, a Homo sapiens design which is widespread among reasonably complex animal forms which undergo development. Thus, the only proper conceptual locale for this idea of the repetition compulsion is the conception of a development which is natural to a neurologically intact member of Homo sapiens in interaction with his or her expectable milieu. This also means that the fact of a repetition compulsion ought not to be recruited into the service of still another, different set of ideas, which are the life and death instincts. These life and death instincts are not motives but are different principles of mental function—opposed ways in which the "psychical apparatus" (Freud, 1900a, p. 540) can be used with regard to psychic tension—and as such can be complexly related to behavior or experience evident in a repetition compulsion. Indeed, Freud (1920g) himself, in the *Beyond the Pleasure Principle* monograph, gives examples of how the repetition compulsion can involve tension maintenance and even increase, as well as tension reduction.

I believe it is correct to say that Freud (1911b) never explicitly attempted to coordinate his earlier, energy-discharge hallucination theory about the origin of meaning (thought) with his later (Freud, 1920c) writing, which now amounted to a genuinely dual principle of mental functioning (Loewald, 1973). It is at least possible to see a hint of such coordination in Freud's (1911b) early work on the origins of thought in the following passage.

> Restraint upon motor discharge . . . was provided by means of the process of *thinking* . . . Thinking was *endowed with characteristics* which made it possible for the mental apparatus to tolerate an increased tension . . . while the process of discharge was postponed. . . . For this purpose the conversion of freely displaceable cathexes into 'bound' cathexis was necessary, *and this was brought about by means of raising the level of the whole cathectic process.* (p. 221, second and third italics mine).

Be this as it may, thought requires for its emergence a principle of mental function which uses psychic tension for the construction of meaning structures. Clinically healthy development into even more mature meaning organization obviously, then, will require a continuous application of psychic tension for the construction of "thought structures" (Freud, 1920a, p. 542). *I can now understand splitting to be an organization of consciousness instigated by psychopathology which is a pathological "compulsion to repeat"* (Freud 1920g, p. 19) *the use of immature meaning structure (function and content) in a core area of self and object representations which govern emotional esteem, survival, and the like.* Therefore, splitting cannot ever be regarded as clinically healthy or be related to psychic system terminology. Splitting always is a miscarriage of psychic structure (function and content), and splitting pertains to a point in the life cycle of such immature pre-Oedipal psychic organization that what we mean by psychic systems simply does not yet exist.

But I trust I have made clear how I believe it would be incorrect to apply any motive-like concept, the "predicate . . . instinctual" (Freud, 1920g, p. 36), to this repetitive, pathological maintenance of immature meaning structure, function, and content, which I believe is splitting. For that matter, I trust I have made it clear that I believe it equally incorrect to talk about psychic development as if it, also, involved a psychoanalytically understood drive or motive.[4] Certainly the entire conglomerate of conflict, the ontogeny of libidinal and aggressive drives with emergent anxieties which Freud (e.g., 1926d) taught us to understand, all of this is part and parcel of the development every human will undergo given expectable circumstances (Hartmann, 1939). But that each human will undergo such a characteristic development is something Homo sapiens shares with all other organisms, each of whom have their own species-characteristic development. This occurs because of how we are designed—made—and ought not to be confused with any sort of psychoanalytically formulated concept of motivation. A human will in time walk upright and, as well, learn an ontogenetically predisposed series of "thought structures" (Freud, 1900a, p. 542) because of how we are made. Also because of how we, like other reasonably complex animals, are made, pathology can prevent such development and can result instead in unproductive repetition.

But now, having located splitting as consciousness mediated by repetition compulsion in an area of immature meaning structure, function, and content, I must turn to a direct examination of how we learn to think and its relevance for our psychoanalytic concepts of splitting and denial (disavowal).

3

The Emergence and Growth of a Meaning Apparatus

I now will take up certain characteristics as to how we think—that is, represent, produce meaning—and especially what this is like for a young (pre-Oedipal into early latency) child. Essentially, this will be an explication of Piaget's (e.g., 1924, 1932, 1936, 1941, 1945, 1947, 1964) work. But I will examine Piaget's work in such a way as to enable a later useful application of Piaget's research to our own psychoanalytic concepts of splitting and denial (disavowal). First I will examine in some detail a number of characteristics as to how young children think. Then I will examine the consequences of how a young child thinks for the way in which a young child can and cannot construct a grade in his or her existence between experience indexed in some way to be real and experience which is in some way not-real.

We owe especially to Piaget an understanding of how the thought structures of young children possess characteristics which make for a unique organization that is discontinuous from the organization of experience mediated by later, mature representation. This difference cannot be grasped by any simple application of terms like "concrete" versus "abstract," which is so often found in the literature (e.g., Jacobson, 1964; Hartmann, 1939). Representations are structures which function for the young child just as they do for a mature adult; that is, representations (concepts) increase predictability in a way that supplements information obtained through perception (Sokolov, 1963). More is known about an object that can be referred to an already formed concept for meaning (Nelson 1974). And, of course, concepts can evoke meaningful experience which does not depend upon immediate perception (e.g., Fraiberg, 1969). But while all of this is true, the immature child does not possess an authentic concept in any conventional, adult sense of the term. Piaget (e.g., 1945) calls these immature thought structures in the young child "preconcepts" (p. 221) and illustrates how uniquely they perform a referential function with examples like the following:

> Piaget is walking along the road with his young daughter Jacqueline (J.), age 2 years, 7 months, 2 days.
>
> She used the term "the slug" for the slugs we went to see every morning along a certain road. At 2, 7, (2) she cried: "There it is!" on seeing one, and . . . when we saw another ten yards further on she said: "There's the slug

> again." I answered: "But isn't it another one?" J. then went back to see the first one. [Piaget says:] "Is it the same one?—"Yes."—Another slug?"—"Yes." "Another or the same?—. . ." The question obviously had no meaning for J. (p. 225)

Another illustration is taken from Jacqueline ten days later while she looks at a photograph of her sister Lucienne (L.) in a new bathing suit.

> J. asks: "*What's the baby's name?*" Her mother explained that it was a bathing costume, but J. pointed to L. herself and said: "But what's the name of that?" [indicating L.'s face] and repeated the question several times. But as soon as L. had her dress on again, J. exclaimed very seriously: "*It's Lucienne again,*" as if her sister had changed her identity in changing her clothes. (p. 224)

A final brief excerpt, a day later, from an example used by Piaget, illustrates the manner in which such an immature representational apparatus performed reference for self-representation.

> Similarly, when I showed J. another photograph of herself, she said: "*It's Jacqueline.*" "Is it you or not?" [Piaget asked.] "Yes, it's me, but what has the Jacqueline in the photo got on her head?" (p. 225)

Piaget (1945) concludes from such observation, and from lifelong work, that preconceptual thought structures possess the following characteristics:

> On the one hand, the particular objects involved in the child's thoughts have less individuality, i.e., they are less identical with themselves, than in the later stages. For instance, . . . J. refused to accept the identity of her sister L. when she was wearing a bathing suit, and then said, "It's Lucienne again," when she was wearing her dress again. J. separated herself, according to the images she saw of herself, into "J. in the glass," "J. doing that," and "J. in the photo." (p. 226)
>
> But on the other hand, classes are less comprehensive than they will be later, *class being a kind of typical individual reproduced in several copies.* Slugs . . . are all "the slug" reappearing in various forms. . . ." (p. 226 italics mine)
>
> These two characteristics, absence of individual identity and of general class, are in reality one and the same. It is because the stable general class does not exist, that the individual elements, not being assembled within the framework of a real whole, partake directly of one another without permanent individuality, and it is the lack of individuality in the parts which prevents the whole from becoming an inclusive class. (p. 226)

There are a number of important considerations about the structure of childish thought which flow from such observations, and which will be shown later to have relevance for the psychoanalytic concepts of splitting and denial (disavowal). Self and object representation structures which are organized as preconcepts always structure meaning about mental content which has perceptual quality, or perceptual-like quality, which inheres in some concrete attribute or action of an inanimate object, oneself, or others (e.g., a bathing suit versus the dress). It is because of this that an *image*-representation naturally arises as the first symbolic vehicle for meaning. We do not deal here simply with a question of the extent to which image versus language functions as a symbolic vehicle of thought. An adult, of course, may use an image for the expression of some idea, but such an image is *fully differentiated as a symbol from the authentic, general class concept which it signifies.* This is not the case with the young child. Further, while a young child will, of course, use a word to communicate an idea to another, any sort of sensitive observation will reveal that it is really a sensorial, concrete, often action-saturated image which actually is being used by the child for the meaning of the idea. ("What is a hole?" "A hole is to dig.")

What is not so easy to grasp, even with sensitive observation, and what is Piaget's (e.g., 1945) significant contribution, is the young child's lack of a full differentiation of the elements of a mature meaning system. One can liken such a mature meaning system to a flower which is destined, given an average expectable environment (Hartmann, 1939), to mature into a three-petaled blossom (see, for example, Ogden and Richards, 1943). The "center petal" will become the authentic class concept. It will possess a stability (e.g., Piaget, 1945) which inheres in its generality (abstractness); that is, it is a meaning structure which functions according to a principle such that it is cognized as a constant *arrangement* of perceptual material from diverse sensory inputs, and this can actually be quite disparate from one experience to another. The "second petal" will become the symbolic vehicle (language, image, or gesture), which will be fully differentiated from the concept, and from the "third petal," which is the particular exemplar of the concept.

The meaning structure of the young child is not such a fully differentiated organization; but neither is it completely undifferentiated like an infant so that, for example, a word is "known" only as an actual property of a thing. The meaning organization of the young child is somewhere in between. It is like a three-petaled blossom which has just begun to differentiate into three leaves. This means that, to the young child, the image-representation performs a kind of "double-duty" and occupies a unique status. The image-representation performs the referential function and evokes perceptually absent experiences as is accomplished by the mature, authentic class concept. But because this childish representation is not yet fully differentiated as a symbol from the class concept, the image itself is cognized as a sort of *prototype picture* for the production of meaning (all slugs are "the slug"). And because the image-representation is not yet fully differentiated as a symbolic vehicle from its referent, the prototype-image continues a "*participation*" (Piaget, 1945, p. 226, italics mine) in the existence of the thing or relation. But one can, indeed must, say, with Piaget, that "participation" also applies to relations among the referents of a preconcept. Each exemplar of a preconcept, while actually a unique and particular entity, cannot be known as such because an immature prototype image-representation agglutinates all meaning to it. It would be as if one were watching a regiment of foot soldiers, composed actually, of course, of different individuals. But in observing this regiment, one could only see the regimental flag-bearer (of meaning), and there is no perception of the actual presence of other soldiers in the regiment (who constitute individual, different exemplars of the authentic class concept). Further, and inevitably, there is no understanding that there exists an unseen regimental command structure (the authentic class concept itself).[1] Piaget (1945) puts it this way:

> The pre-concept involves the image and is partially determined by it, whereas the concept, precisely because of its generality, breaks away from the image and uses it only as an illustration. (p. 229)
>
> Thus, "the slug" is the prototype or representative of all slugs, while in a general concept all slugs are equivalent through their common abstract characteristics. Hence the particular image to which "the slug" corresponds keeps a much higher value, with respect to other slugs, than the equally particular image which serves as individual symbol to a [latency age] child [now] thinking in terms of the general class of slugs. (p. 228)

Piaget's comprehension of the structure of childish meaning is no mere logical analysis. It is a significant contribution to our understanding of the "psychical apparatus" (Freud, 1900, p. 538) and how immaturity in this apparatus partly determines experience and behavior. We can now understand that the young child makes meaning that is magical—but naively magical. What one, paradoxically, can call "real" magic is a *conscious intention* to treat a prototype image symbol *as if* it is not yet fully differentiated from its referent, so that it continues a "participation" (Piaget, 1945, p. 226) in the existence of this referent. Then, by a magical word, or a voodoo doll, or a gesture, etc., the magician "expects" to control in some manner the thing or person so represented. With the young child, it is an innocent (that is, unknowing) magic, which inheres in the way he or she makes meaning.[2] Also, and I repeat, the young child's ideas center about impelling, perceptual-like qualities of self and object representation, or motor-like qualities (e.g., kinesthesis), which inhere in actions connected with referents, so it is natural that prototype *imagery* be used to organize such immature preconcepts. This means that, at best, childish ideas communicated in language are like some guest uncomfortable in a house ill-designed to the child's needs. As Piaget (1945) puts it, "these half-general, half-individual schemas . . . constitute pre-concepts [and] the word or collective sign is still inadequate to the content of these. . . ." (p. 228) Vivid visual, or visual-like quality, smell, touch, kinesthesis, taste, etc., are more faithfully expressed with gesture, action, and drawing. I also can cite A. Freud's (1968) observation that for all young children "not thought or speech but *motor actions* are their legitimate media of expression and communication" (p. 169, italics mine). If one understands in this statement that "thought or speech" refer to two different ingredients of a mature meaning apparatus, then such observation based upon psychoanalytic practice becomes congruent with Piaget's conclusions about the inadequacy of language for the expression of preconceptual thought. That two such very different methodologies produce a similar interpretation about the nature of an immature meaning apparatus constitutes especially powerful evidence for the acceptance of such a conclusion. And A. Freud's (1968) further conclusion that such a natural, childish expression of immature thought in activity should not be confused with "acting out" (p. 169) is pertinent not only to the treatment of children but also for narcissistic and borderline adults, who, I will later show, continue to possess and operate on the basis of such an immature meaning apparatus.

Further, the way the young child organizes meaning with preconcepts produces a special, immature consequence for social experience, that is, for the representation of a relationship between self and others. Piaget's term for this is "egocentricity" (e.g., 1947), but it might better be termed "noncentricity." Since preconcepts are always "centered" (Piaget, 1945, p. 235) on some particular, striking perceptual or motor-like qualities of some entity, an interpersonal relationship can only mean to a young child something which is immediately, subjectively evident; and such knowledge cannot include another, different viewpoint. The young child knows there is a *bodily* other who is not the self. But any representation of the bodily other's *experience* can only be in terms of the child's own immediate experience. As Piaget (1947) puts it, the young child refers the experience of the other "to his point of view" (p. 160) and therefore distorts without realizing it because the child "cannot yet distinguish his point of view from that of others through failure to coordinate [differentiate and integrate into one meaning structure] the points of view" (p. 160). Paradoxically, but understandably, because a child cannot structure such a coordination and integration of points of view, the child actually (objectively) may become "centered" (Piaget 1945, p. 235) upon the experience of the other, so that a young child is especially susceptible to imitation and suggestion. But again, such suggestion and imitation have no meaning for the child in terms of any knowledge of another's viewpoint. Piaget (e.g., 1947) often has pointed out how young children will not understand that their own imitation is imitation, but will believe instead that they have originated such behavior. Social experience has no meaning for young children in terms of complementary or supplementary roles; their meaning apparatus does not enable it, and this is congruent with Kernberg's (1966) conclusion that an organization of social experience in terms of roles is indicative of the acquisition of mature identification structures.

The immature meaning apparatus of the young child also has a significant consequence for the way the young child reasons. Because the young child has no stable class concept, neither authentic deductive nor inductive part-whole reasoning is possible. But the young child does reason, and it is important to understand how this is accomplished. Piaget's special term for how the young child does reason is "transduction" (e.g., 1945, p. 234). The young child interrelates his or her preconcepts by a kind of direct, qualitative connection of experiences, one to the other. The young child reasons from particular to particular, producing or obtaining meaning from some salient or impelling aspect of some initial event and irreversibly drawing a conclusion to some other consequence, and again on the basis of some perceptual or motor impelling aspect of the occurrence.

Finally, there is something which I believe I can later show to have a direct pertinence to psychoanalytic concepts of splitting and denial (disavowal). It is also at once clear how this immature meaning apparatus must produce a special relationship between experience indexed by the young child to be "actual" (not play) and that which carries some type of notation of "not-real" (play). I have indicated that a fundamental characteristic of a young child's preconceptual thought has to do with how a prototype image-representation continues a "participation" (Piaget, 1945, p. 226) in the existence of the referent so connoted by the representation. And I have indicated how magic is nothing else but a conscious intention to treat some symbolic vehicle as able through such participation to control the thing so represented. When young children are at play, they are not engaged in any such intentional magic. Actually, young children cannot comprehend magic, if we mean by it a regression in the meaning apparatus in the service of the ego (Kris, 1952) such that the symbolic vehicle is treated as if it had participation in the referent's existence. But it is the same potentiality for adult magic which is inherent in the structure of childish thought. I believe this is congruent with what A. Freud (1936) has called a "hypercathexis of . . . fantasy," (p. 81) and which she understands to be characteristic of childish play. This "hypercathexis of . . . fantasy" (A. Freud, 1936, p. 81) is enabled in part because with a child, without conscious intention, an image-representation continues to participate in the existence of the referent.

Then, inasmuch as the content of the preconceptual identificatory structure always involves some impelling perceptual, kinesthetic, auditory, etc., quality, all the young child need do is express such qualities and he or she "becomes" the thing or person in play. A little boy or girl, say, can put on a cowboy or a cowgirl costume and "become" a cowboy or a cowgirl. Piaget (1945) puts it this way:

> What is, in fact, the difference between the act of . . . separating oneself into several characters, or reducing several slugs into one, and that of identifying in

> play one object with another and oneself with other people? Is it not merely that in one case there is *belief* and an effort in adaptation, and in the other case there is only *pretense* and assimilation. . . . Apart from this functional distinction, the pre-concept and the ludic [i.e., playful] symbol both proceed . . . by pre-logical "participation." (p. 227, italics mine)

Of course, we are all familiar with even more extreme assimilating behavior and experience which can characterize childish play. All that a young child need do is pick up a twig, thrust it vigorously straight up into the air, and an astronaut is on a flight to the moon. All that a young child need do is to ride a bike, hard and fast, and some heroic self-representation can become playfully alive. Such is the imaginative world children can construct by playfully enlivening what are actually everyday, mundane features of their world, and they can do this by extreme assimilation of such everyday material to prototype image-representation.

In play, as A. Freud (1936) puts it, a child is "insensible of . . . reality" (p. 80). But what Piaget's (e.g., 1945) work makes clear is that such "insensibility" is enabled in part by the way young children naturally produce meaning, and this same meaning structure and function apply to adaptive as well as playful behavior and experience. Piaget (1924) puts it as follows:

> Actually, play cannot [in the young child] be opposed to reality, because in both cases belief is arbitrary and pretty much destitute of logical reasons. Play is a reality which the child is disposed to believe in when by himself, just as reality is a game at which he is willing to play with the adult and anyone else who believes in it. . . .Thus we have to say of child play that it constitutes an autonomous reality, but with the understanding that the 'true' reality to which it is opposed is considerably less "true" for the child than for us. (Cited in Flavell [1963], p. 161)

But it is a serious mistake to conclude from this that a clinically healthy child does not accommodate to changing *actualities* in his or her life. I use the term "actualities" because I need to find and use some term other than "reality."[3] I will reserve the term "reality" for use only in a context wherein the meaning apparatus has achieved a structural differentiation between experience which is indexed as not-real and that which is indexed as real, and I believe this is not the case until sometime in mid-latency (Steingart, 1969). Nevertheless, the clinically healthy young child *functionally* will accommodate to actual, impelling changes in his or her life circumstance with a natural relinquishment of some assimilating, playful self or object representation in favor of adaptive behavior when this becomes necessary. Let a clinically healthy young child be absorbed in some outdoors, grandiose, heroic play as an astronaut, or whatever; then the sky suddenly darkens while there occurs some frightening clap of thunder, and the same child will naturally foresake such play for the experienced safety, comfort, and protection of home and mother. Such an observation can be multiplied endlessly, and is commonplace; but for that it is not the less significant. In this sense, clinically healthy children are supremely responsive to actuality, *and this arises from the same characteristics of an immature meaning apparatus.*

It is not only that such alternation in the behavior of a clinically healthy young child is an "inconsistency which has no disturbing effect." (A. Freud, 1936, p. 80). It is precisely this kind of natural flux between assimilating play and meaning accommodated to actualities which is the hallmark of clinical health at this point in the life cycle. I already have indicated how this same meaning apparatus also will produce, unknowingly, extreme accommodating responses in the form of gross imitation by the clinically healthy young child. For example, think for a moment how a clinically healthy young child can assiduously and laboriously copy a drawing of some object to the utmost detail of which he or she is capable. In fact, as Piaget's (e.g., 1945) work makes clear, the development of thought in young children into adaptive, mature representational structures can be described as a continuous, functionally fluid interaction and eventual integration of such assimilating and accommodating activities.

It is, of course, especially Winnicott (e.g., 1951) who introduced into our literature the importance of play, not only for normal development but for a viable treatment process as well. However, as important as I consider Winnicott's contribution to be about these matters, I also believe that a certain corrective has to be introduced into his formulations. Thus, I don't believe one can say "Play belongs to the. . .theoretical line between the subjective and that which is objectively perceived" (Winnicott, 1951, p. 50). Young children simply do not "objectively perceive" in any case, if we mean by this a meaning organization which differentiates experience indexed as real versus not-real, such as is possible for a late latency child (Steingart, 1969). But a clinically healthy young child will adaptively adjust playful, grandiose, and idealizing meanings about self or others in response to changing actualities which require that this be done.

I now have described something of the way in which young children represent—that is, how they acquire and make meaning. Also, I have indicated how the preconceptual meaning structures of young children implicate a special status from prototype image-representation. This, in turn, has a profound consequence for our proper understanding of the language of young children, their social experience, reasoning, and also most especially for the way in which the clinically healthy young child can functionally, but not structurally, establish a flexible vicissitude between play and changing actualities in his or her life. This meaning apparatus itself emerges from an earlier sensory-motor intelligence, and out of such a childish meaning apparatus there will emerge in normal development, with an average expectable environment (Hartmann, 1939), other kinds of representational capabilities with entirely different characteristics. I have detailed elsewhere (Steingart, 1969) these later kinds of representation-making capabilities. I will now again, briefly at least, describe these acquisitions because they are relevant to later aspects of this investigation.

Briefly, then, the meaning structures which emerge out of childish, preconceptual thought Piaget (e.g., 1947) calls "concrete operations" (p. 123), and this is achieved in mid-latency. By implication, I already have indicated the significant change in intellect achieved with "concrete operations": A meaning structure now emerges which possesses a full differentiation among idea, symbolic vehicle, and referent (thing, other, relation); a representation itself now possesses the stableness characteristic of a mature, general, abstract concept. Piaget (e.g., 1947) refers to this stableness characteristic of a mature concept with such terms as "conservation," (p. 140) or "grouping," (p. 142) or "mobile equilibrium" (p. 142). It means, for example, that now the concept of a "slug" is abstractly or generally applicable to each and every instance of a perceived, particular slug, *but is none of these,* so that each particular slug retains its own, actual, particular identity (Piaget, 1945). Or, for example, a quantity of liquid which is objectively the same amount will be known to be equivalent even though perceptual appearances may be dramatically changed by placement of identical quantities in very differently shaped containers (Piaget, 1941, cited in Hunt, 1961). Such stableness in representation can, of course, carry over to self and object representation and then will be a determinant of mature personality organization (Steingart, 1969).

There is a final representational capability which can appear in adolescence that is termed by Piaget (e.g., 1947) "formal operations" (p. 137). The intelligence of a person who utilizes "formal operations" has been called by Piaget (1964) "thought raised to the second power" (p. 63). While, says Piaget (1964),"concrete thinking is the representation of a possible action . . . formal thinking is the representation of a representation of a possible action" (p. 63). The significance of this acquisition is that all ideas are now known as human inventions and not somehow produced in the flux of concrete experience. For example, an adolescent can grasp a concept which intrinsically can never be secured in some concrete experience, such as the idea of infinity. This same knowledge, that a representation is a human creation, also can apply to any meaning which is the content of self or object representation.

4

On the Concept of a Meaning Disturbance—Pathological Play

The previous material now can be used to develop the concept of a meaning disturbance as pathological play. This idea of a meaning disturbance will be seen to include what is clinically relevant for the concept of splitting and, as well, provides a basis for relating this notion of splitting to the concept of denial (disavowal). This concept of a meaning disturbance places a proper weight upon a disturbance in reality appraisal, which should be understood to be something which always occurs when an individual employs splitting and denial. Inasmuch as a meaning disturbance does involve psychopathology in reality appraisal, it is not a neurotic phenomenon. But a meaning disturbance does not involve a schizophrenic reconstruction of reality (hallucination or delusion). Thus, a meaning disturbance is a distinct type of psychopathology which is neither neurotic nor schizophrenic.

All that I have discussed thus far has to do with the age expectable development of psychic structure in general, and of a meaning apparatus in particular, given an average expectable environment (Hartman, 1939). But have I said anything about the psychoanalytic concepts of splitting and denial (disavowal)? I think not. But a path between the way clinically healthy young children make meaning, and the psychoanalytic concepts of splitting and denial, can be created in three steps.

The first step is the realization (something that only could have been provided by psychoanalysis) that there exists a developmental series of qualities presented to a young child's experience simply because he or she is a human. Gross psychic pleasure itself versus gross psychic pain is, of course, a fundamental, impelling difference in experience from a psychoanalytic point of view. But beyond this, our theories of psychosexual development (e.g., Freud, 1905d), as well as our theories about the development of narcissism (e.g., Freud, 1914c; Kohut, 1971) and object relations (e.g., Freud, 1910h; Mahler, 1968; Kernberg,1966) cannot help but also be at the same time statements about a further differentiation and integration of psychic pleasures or pains which are presented to the child's experience. Such an unfolding of psychic pleasures and pains not only has a pertinence to drives, or narcissism, or object relationships, it also *provides data* for a meaning apparatus; and such data will be processed according to procedures for representation with respect to how the apparatus works at any period in development. A young child, who naturally represents preconcepts with prototype images which are centered upon some impelling feature of a referent, will naturally come to structure representations in terms of some such impelling difference in psychic pleasure and pain qualities. This is hardly a new idea. I already have mentioned that Freud (1915c), almost seventy years ago, described how the young child will naturally use pleasure versus pain qualities as the basis for an initial representation of self versus not-self areas of experience, and he did so without once using the idea of splitting. I already have suggested elsewhere (Steingart, 1969) that an immature, narcissistic "self love," once described by Freud (1914c), is another kind of special, unfolding, impelling, pleasure prototype image-representation, and that the later mature integration of this representation is critical for character formation (see also Stolorow and Lachmann, 1980). An epigenetic documentation of how narcissistic-, drive-, and object-relationship-connected psychic pleasure and pain qualities contribute data for representation to the young child's meaning apparatus, and of the stages which lead to an integration of immature self and object representations into maturely structured concepts, is an important future theoretical task. Obviously self and object representation must go beyond a preconcept centering on various qualities of psychic pleaure and pain if this is to take place. But I consider that Piaget's (e.g., 1945) work makes clear that we deal here with no simple line of succession. Certainly we can consider that self and object representation content related to narcissistic, object-relations, and drive pleasures and pains are, for psychoanalysis, *primus inter pares.* But the young child is, at the same time, busily building up such representational structures centered about a variety of impelling sensory and motor qualities (that is, other than psychic pleasures and pains). Freud (1915c) once hypothesized as to how an immature procedure for the construction of a set of representations, "inside" versus "outside", was based upon whether some experienced stimulation was made to cease by virtue of one's own activity.[1]

Piaget's investigations thus fit well with Hartmann's (1939) work. The meaning apparatus is no different in this respect from any apparatus, say, the motor apparatus. The meaning apparatus has an autonomous origin (Hartmann 1939). It is not drive-created, but certainly drive-, narcissistic-, and object-relations-connected at every point of the life cycle. We deal always with a matter of relative autonomy which makes for clinical health or pathology. I consider that it is not in keeping with observation to formulate any sort of progression which initiates representation with self and object representations only centered about psychic pleasures and pains.

But this matter of a relative autonomy of the meaning apparatus from drive, narcissistic, and object-relationship dynamics brings us to the second step toward the psychoanalytic concepts of splitting and denial. Again, the meaning apparatus is no different in this respect from any other apparatus, say, the motor.

The motor apparatus may function with insufficient autonomy from drive, narcissistic, or object-relationship conflicts. Just as we know that immature motor behavior can be used to avoid what would otherwise develop into conflictual experience, so can an immature meaning apparatus be used for the same purpose. I thus understand splitting and denial to be a use of an immature, preconcept, prototype image representation meaning apparatus in a core area of self and object representation, as a defense against conflictual experience. I stress that splitting and denial is the maintenance of an immature meaning apparatus in what I call a "core area" of self and object representation; that is, it is directly related to self and object esteem and/or survival, because it is this which implicates conflictual experience. Clinically, it is commonplace to observe how, with respect to both adults and children, representational structures can continue to mature outside of such a core area of self and object representation. It belongs to such a conception that when an immature meaning apparatus is used for such a defensive purpose, no further development of meaning can take place in this core area of self and object representation. The representation-making apparatus within this core area of self and object representation no longer is importantly effected by a principle of mental function (Freud, 1920g, 1924c) which implements psychic tension for the further development of meaning structures; instead the meaning apparatus now operates essentially according to a mental principle of psychic function which makes representation for a reduction or elimination of psychic tension.

The third step toward the realization of these psychoanalytic concepts of splitting and denial involves their relationship to each other. Freud (1927e) first explicitly interrelated these two terms in his explanation of fetishism, but there is no consensus in subsequent literature about this matter. For example, the term "splitting" does not even appear in the subject index of Jacobson's (1964) *Self and Object World* monograph, nor is it explicitly used in her important theoretical paper on "Denial and Repression" (Jacobson, 1957). But splitting is certainly implied in statements by her like the following: "structural conflicts are thus replaced by conflicts between opposing instinctual strivings which. . .may be alternately used to deny and screen each other" (Jacobson, 1975, p. 108). But other writers go beyond an omission, or a lack of interrelationship with regard to these two terms, and specifically argue that the connection between splitting and denial is not as simple and straightforward as Freud described it. What is interesting, but also confusing, is that these arguments—that there exists a more complex relationship between splitting and denial—go in two opposite directions in our literature. Certain writers (Stewart, 1970; Trunnel and Holt, 1974) argue that splitting can occur in varying contexts of personality organization and function, so that it does not necessarily implicate a denial of reality consideration such as Freud (1940a) described in the *Outline*. Kernberg (1975a), on the other hand, refers the concept of denial to a continuum of personality organization and function, and apparently equates a least-integrated kind of denial with splitting. Kernberg (1975a) states, "Denial, then, is a broad *group* of defensive operations . . . related at its higher level to isolation and other higher level defenses . . . and at its lower level to splitting" (p. 32–33, italics mine). I believe it is certain that at least part of the reason for this current inconsistency or omission in the use of these two terms is a legacy from Freud's own writing. I will examine Freud's writing shortly, as well as literature subsequent to Freud which bears upon this matter. But I first will identify my own relationship to Freud's writing, and then show how a meaning apparatus orientation brings about theoretical clarification.

I will adhere to Freud's final formulation about this matter. In Freud's (1940a) unfinished *Outline*, he stated the following:

> The disavowal is always supplemented by an acknowledgement; two contradictory and independent attitudes always arise and result in the situation of there being a splitting of the ego. (p. 204)

And, in Freud's (1940e) unfinished "Splitting of the Ego in the Process of Defense," he said as follows:

> With the help of certain mechanisms he *rejects reality* . . . [but] on the other hand, in the same breath he recognizes the danger of *reality* . . . (p. 275, italics mine)

Then Freud added:

> Everything has to be paid for . . . and this success is achieved at the price of a . . . splitting of the ego. (p. 275–276)

An immediate question, and problem, which arises is Freud's use of a concept "ego" in this context. My earlier general comments about the relationship between a psychoanalytic concept of self and our psychic system terminology, together with Hartmann's (1950) realization that Freud did not always explicitly distinguish in his writing between the term "ego" as a psychic system and self representation as mental content, apply to this question. I believe we can and should reread these statements by Freud to mean that splitting and denial have to do with an immature period of personality development. And during this early period in the life cycle, the organization of consciousness, which includes this matter of a notation of real from not-real experience, will in part be determined by features of an immature meaning apparatus. That Freud himself, at least at one time, considered such a meaning apparatus orientation is clear from a statement from his Fetishism (1927e) paper. Freud stated:

> I also began to suspect that [such] occurrences [i.e., splitting and denial] . . . in childhood are by no means rare . . . (p. 156)

An adult, added Freud, possesses

> *a higher degree of differentiation in the psychical apparatus*; things might be permissible to a child which could entail severe injury to an adult. (p. 156, italics mine)

Looked at from a meaning apparatus perspective, the necessity for an intrinsic relationship between splitting and denial (disavowal) now at once becomes clear, inasmuch as both splitting and denial simply touch upon different aspects of the same pathological use of an immature meaning apparatus which is natural to early childhood.

Recall that this immature "symbolic function" (Piaget, 1945, p. 278) has these fundamental characteristics:

(1) A mature conceptual construction for self and object representation does not exist. Discrete, actually unique and individual referents (things, persons, relations) are not known as such, each show "participation" (Piaget, 1951, p. 226) readily with each other, and so lack individuality; each will lose any discrete, stable content enabled by reference to an authentically mature conceptual structure. Thus, for example, a prototype-image self or object representation which is idealized, "bad," "good," or whatever can agglutinate to it for meaning what are actually (objectively) exemplar entities or aspects that differ from each other. *It is the pathological misuse of these attributes of an immature meaning apparatus which I can now define as a psychoanalytic concept of splitting.* This, loosely, might be considered the content aspect of the pathological misuse of an immature meaning apparatus.

(2) Preconcepts altogether, including their articulation as vivid self and object prototype-image representations, are not fully differentiated as such from their referents (things, persons, relations), *and what results from this is a notation of belief.* For example, self and object representations which may possess impelling, grandiose, and idealized content (e.g., Freud, 1914c; Kohut, 1971) will carry belief for the young child. This is because all preconceptual representations possessed by the young child are known in such a way as to possess a "participation" (Piaget, 1951, p. 226) in the actuality of those referents (people, things, relations) for which they provide meaning. *It is the pathological misuse of this attribute of an immature meaning apparatus which I now define as denial, and which I think carries a simple and straightforward implication for a disturbance in reality appraisal.*

A striking clinical example of such pathological meaning production is provided by Jacobson (1957) in her important paper "Denial and Repression." A male analysand is described for whom any guilty feelings or thoughts meant the presence on his wife's face of a "reproachful and hurt look" (Jacobson, 1957, p. 126). This man then would attempt to make this hurt and reproachful look disappear by producing "an expression [via sex, etc.] of delight on her face" (Jacobson, 1957, p. 126), and in so doing, the man himself no longer experienced (knew) guilt. At the same time, this man could hurt his wife "by rather cruel remarks, but was quite unaware of his behavior" (Jacobson, 1957, p. 118); that is, so long as there did not appear on the wife's face a hurt, reproachful look. Certainly, the etiology and dynamics of this "reproachful and hurt look" (Jacobson, 1957, p. 126) were examined in the analysis: The look first was "seen" on the face of a pregnant toad after the analysand, as a young boy, sadistically tortured the toad and then killed the animal in order to "make it [the look] . . . disappear" (Jacobson, 1957, p. 114). This pregnant toad torture and murder occurred at a time the boy's mother was pregnant—pregnant, of course, with a future rival and impregnated by a rival father. The mother subsequently miscarried this baby, aspects of which most likely were witnessed by the child. The mother lapsed into a depression for many weeks following this miscarriage. The boy, confusingly, held himself responsible via his "depressive reproachful mother [who] appeared to blame him forever" (Jacobson, 1957, p. 115), experienced the bloody miscarriage as evidence of his mother's castrated state, and so forth. But the thrust of Jacobson's (1957) paper is to consider how this man "*conceived* of . . . psychic manifestations . . . as if they were concrete" (p. 125, italics mine), so that, for example, a guilty versus praiseworthy self-representation content could be realized directly by the appearance of reproach or delight on his wife's face. Jacobson (1957) proposes that this presupposes "an infantile concretization of psychic reality which permits persons . . . to treat their psychic strivings as if they were concrete objects *perceived*" (p. 125, italics mine). However, from the perspective of an immature meaning apparatus, one can state this in another way which I believe adds clarity. There certainly is no issue here of perception which replaces thought (conception), which would only be the case with hallucination. Rather, it is a matter of an immature thought (meaning production) apparatus which is opera-tive in a core area of representation which governs self and object esteem and/or survival; what an experience in this core area will mean will be determined in part by some prototype-image (reproachful face versus delighted face, etc.) which agglutinates all experience relevant to it, and this image-representation (like all imagery) will be saturated with sensory and motor qualities.

With regard to the case material (Jacobson, 1957) to which I have just alluded, one can say that a notation of belief necessarily adhered to such guilt content such that it became imperative that the analysand do something to make such guilt (the reproachful look) disappear. This can be called the formal aspect of a pathological misuse of an immature meaning apparatus. But I repeat and stress that these formal and content aspects, splitting and denial, always implicate each other. Splitting and denial are interrelated aspects of the same pathological misuse of the way an immature psychic apparatus produces meaning. *Altogether, I will designate these two interrelated kinds of pathological misuse of an immature meaning apparatus as a meaning disturbance.*

But this term "denial" (disavowal), even though now understood to be belief naturally attached to a pathological misuse of split mental contents produced by an immature meaning apparatus, still only emphasizes such belief in the negative. Denial as a term implies a reality (actuality for the young child) to which a person does not want to attach belief for reasons having to do with dynamic conflict. Therefore, another term is needed to emphasize the "positive," although equally pathological, conscious belief a person can want to attach to immature split mental contents, and for this I can speak about illusion. With respect to the young child, I am now in a position to say that it is the presence of *illusion versus gratifying but also productive play* which discriminates between clinical health and psychopathology. This can be put another way: A meaning disturbance can be described as a (mis)use of cognition as *pathological play* which a young child defensively uses to deny certain actualities, or an adult uses to deny certain realities, and to which have become attached intolerable psychodynamic conflicts.

The point is worth repeating that, in the young child, neither clinically healthy play nor pathological, playful illusion have anything to do with differentiation in the meaning apparatus, which actually structures real from not-real experience. It is, I believe, misleading to describe a young child as someone for whom "reality is acknowledged simultaneously" (Fine, Joseph, and Waldhorn, 1969, p. 48) with his or her play. Piaget (e.g., 1945) puts the matter this way with regard to how the young child attaches belief to his or her experience:

> At the level of early childhood there are two contrasting types [of belief], the one connected with social, and more particularly adult behaviors, the other with spontaneous and egocentric individual behaviors. . . .When the child plays, he certainly does not believe, in the sense of socialized belief, in the content of his symbolism, but precisely because symbolism is egocentric thought we have no reason to suppose that he does not believe *in his own way* anything he chooses. . . .There is no question, therefore, in the early stages of symbolic play, of consciousness of make-believe like that of drama or poetry. The . . . child does not consider whether his ludic [i.e., playful] symbols are real or not. He is aware in a sense that they are not so for others, and makes no serious effort to persuade the adult that they are. But for him it is a question which does not arise, because symbolic play is direct satisfaction . . . and has its own kind of belief. (pp. 167–168)

And, as a footnote to these remarks, Piaget adds the following:

> It is only after the age of seven that play really becomes make-believe in contrast to "reflective belief" [i.e., reality]. (p. 168)

What Piaget here is describing is a clinically healthy child, someone whose playful beliefs have a free and easy relationship with changing actuality. Further, it is often not difficult to observe and document the presence of pathological, playful illusion in a young child. Anna Freud (1936), for example, describes the case of a young child who wanted to act as if he were his father:

> He used to put on his father's hat and walk about in it. As long as nobody interfered with him, he was contented and happy. . . . whenever he was forced to take off the hat, indoors, at meals or when he went to bed, he *reacted with restlessness and ill humor*. . . .The difference between him and the little boy who *plays* at being a big man is simply that my small patient's play was *for earnest* . . . (p. 88, italics mine)

A little boy in psychotherapy with me once told me that "some boys are as strong as men." When I responded with a comment that I could understand that this could be a wish of his, he responded quite earnestly and with some irritation, "No, it's so; not all boys are as strong as men, but some are." Even such very brief clinical materials illustrates how, at least in these episodes, a young child can (mis)use playful, not-real experience to promote a gratifying illusion, something which then functions like a defense against split-off actualities about him or herself which have become intolerable because of psychodynamic conflict.

Thus, according to the conception of splitting developed here, splitting cannot be considered an adaptive pattern in which the "affective coloration of infantile experiences dictates the separate grouping of the memory traces of these experiences (Lichtenberg and Slap, 1973, p. 780). Certainly, such "affective coloration," that is, variety among psychic pleasures and pains, normally is *one among a number* of impelling qualities about which preconceptual meanings become centered, and thus organized. But splitting of mental contents always implicates a pathological misuse of such immature meaning organization. Now, instead of a flexible to and fro among such immature meaning structures characteristic of the clinically healthy young child, we observe behavior from which we infer a rigid, pathological keeping-apart of mental contents for purposes of defense against conflict, with denial and playful illusion in regard to actualities in the child's life.[2] It also follows that splitting is not a "pathological counterpart to . . . synthesis" (Lichtenberg and Slap, 1973, p. 775). Splitting, in a loose descriptive sense, might be described as a pathological form of differentiation if we intend by this simply to stress the rigid character of any sort of defensive process. At this point I believe I am close but not identical to a conception of splitting by Kernberg (1975a) that I already have cited. Kernberg (1975a) states, "This defensive division of the ego, in which what was at first a simple defect in integration is then used actively for other purposes, is in essence the mechanism of splitting" (p. 25). However, Kernberg (1975a) also states "this mechanism [splitting] is *normally* used only in an early stage of *ego* development" (italics mine, p. 25). I have indicated that I believe it is clarifying to speak here not about an "ego" but about self and object representations made by a meaning apparatus which produces preconcept, prototype-image representations. In this way, the usage of the term "ego" is reserved for the psychic system ego, which is a late acquisition and which in part is determined by a mature representational apparatus (Steingart, 1969). Further, splitting could just as well be thought of as a pathological form of integration, inasmuch as both differentiating and integrating processes enter into the construction of any immature meaning structures (just as is true with later developing kinds of mature meaning organizations). I believe the substantive point is this: Splitting (and denial or playful illusion) do not pertain directly to those processes of differentiation and integration which produce the *natural* emergence of immature organizations of representation. Splitting (and denial or playful illusion) do pertain to the pathological misuse made of such immature meaning organizations. This is no different from the way a young child can show a pathological misuse of motor skill which, in itself, had developed in an age-expectable fashion up to a certain point in development. However, once pathologically established, splitting (and denial or playful illusion) will prevent further differentiation and integration (development) into mature meaning organizations in a core area of self and object representation which governs self and object esteem and/or survival. This is a necessary way of stating things whenever one utilizes an emergent-structural theory of development, and psychoanalysis surely is such a theory.[3]

I consider that the framework developed here for a psychoanalytic concept of splitting facilitates inquiry about a related question, whether or not splitting is to be regarded as a normal occurrence in that development of the individual which Mahler (e.g., 1968) terms "individuation" (p. 35). Mahler, Pine, and Bergman (1975) describe how certain children "split the object *more permanently than is optimal* into "good" and "bad" (p. 108, italics mine). Such a statement at least implies a belief that splitting is to be considered a normal feature of individuation. This is congruent with the statement I just cited by Kernberg, who indicates that splitting is "normally used only in an early stage" (1975a, p. 25). But Mahler, Pine, and Bergman (1975) also define splitting in this way: "A defense mechanism *often found* during the rapprochement subphase . . ." (p. 292, italics mine). A statement such as the latter, that splitting is "often found," suggests that splitting is not to be regarded as a regular feature of normal maturation. It may be that no child has ever, or will ever, live who does not use splitting as a defense to some extent. But splitting, as a defensive use of an immature, preconceptual thought apparatus, must be theoretically distinguished from how meaning structures in the young child naturally center about any and all sources of impelling sensory and motor-like qualities for the production of a representation. Therefore, I understand this language, "more permanently than is optimal" (Mahler, Pine, and Bergman, 1975), to be a condensing of clinically normal and psychopathological possibilities, which theoretically should be separated from each other. Also, I would not, therefore, speak about splitting as found "in normal children at an earlier age . . . and in borderline or psychotic patients at a later age'' (Greenspan, 1979, p. 315).

Moreover, I am not convinced by any current clinical observation that has been reported, plus my own experience, that splitting must be considered a regular feature of normal development. This question also relates to the question of whether denial and splitting ought to be considered to be a normal precursor to the establishment of repression, and this has been suggested by various writers (e.g., Jacobson, 1957; Kernberg, 1975a). Jacobson (1957), in particular, has examined this question in a thoughtful paper and argues for a point of view that denial be considered a normal precursor to the establishment of repression. But it is difficult to see how this can be so on conceptual, let alone clinical, grounds. Jacobson (1957) herself emphasizes how ultimately all defenses serve the avoidance of anxiety, but in repression signal anxiety mobilizes a defensive struggle against the sources of the danger, i.e., the instinctual drives'' (p. 120). But then Jacobson (1957) goes on to indicate that what ''seems characteristic of denial [is] that to begin with the ego reacts to the danger signal by an *immediate* attempt to ignore this very [anxiety] signal itself'' (p. 121, italics mine). So how can a defense such as denial, which from the first acts to ignore the very experience of anxiety, be considered to be a normal or natural precursor of repression which exactly is attuned to anxiety as a danger signal? I am inclined to believe that just the opposite is the case than what has been suggested in the literature. That is, that an emphasis upon the use of denial and splitting as a defense in early childhood is precisely what works against the establishment of repression as a defense in later development.

Freud (1915c) once described something he called ''instinctual vicissitudes''(p. 132), and some other comments he made in connection with this now are pertinent:

> We shall be approaching a more general realization—namely, that the instinctual vicissitudes which consist in the instincts being turned round upon subject's own ego and undergoing reversal from activity to passivity are dependent on the . . . organization of the ego. *They correspond to the attempts at defense which at higher stages of development of the ego are affected by other means.* (p. 132, italics mine)

Once again, if we reread ''ego'' in a context of early (pre-Oedipal) childhood to mean that immature, not yet integrated panoply of self-representation sets (Steingart, 1969), then Freud here raises interesting questions which should be answerable by clinical observation. I think it reasonable to suppose that Freud had repression in mind when he spoke about defense at ''higher stages of development.'' If so, then one might expect that, all else being equal, the more use in early childhood of such reversal into passivity, the more repression, to gether with defenses which use repression, at a later point in development. In any event, a prototype self-image centered about quality which has to do with what Freud called "passivity" is certainly a different representation of oneself than one with content focused about "activity." Freud also described in this same paper another instinctual vicissitude wherein the child uses for instinctual gratification part of his or her own body. We can consider that a self representation involved in such an experience is also importantly different in quality from prototype self-images which provide meaning for gratification acquired through either passive or active instinctual involvement with another, or with an inanimate object. I suspect that what is critical for clinical health for the young child is not a matter of whether one or another type of instinctual vicissitude is dominant, but whether the child shows a capability for flexible use of all such vicissitudes. I believe that close, clinical developmental study with such an orientation would be extremely valuable.

5

A Comparative Psychopathology Approach to Splitting and Denial

After having obtained what I believe to be clear and useful conceptions of splitting and denial, as particular kinds of developmental psychopathology which altogether involve a meaning disturbance as pathological play, I will apply this conceptualization of a meaning disturbance to our comparative psychopathology literature. I am, of course, especially interested in literature about borderline and narcissistic personality disorders inasmuch as these ideas of splitting and denial especially are applied to these diagnostic entities. But, in addition, I use the particular concepts of splitting and denial I have developed to order a relationship between borderline and narcissistic personalities and the other major diagnostic entities, including clinically healthy behavior and experience. First, I will examine closely Freud's writings on the concepts of splitting and denial (disavowal), as well as examining subsequent literature related to his writings. Later I will take up the Kohut-Kernberg controversy (e.g., Ornstein, 1978; Kernberg, 1974; Kernberg, 1975a; Kernberg, 1975b; Kohut, 1971, 1977) about how to understand and treat narcissistic disturbance, and suggest a resolution which derives from the manner in which I have conceptualized splitting and denial (disavowal) as a meaning disturbance which can be likened to pathological play.

Stewart (1970) puts his finger on an important problem which is one source of confusion surrounding Freud's writing about the concept of splitting, and asks an important question: Can any formulation of Freud's about the idea of splitting, written before the still to be developed structural viewpoint, be the same as what Freud later meant by splitting once he had conceptualized a mature personality as an organization composed of id, ego, and superego subsystems? Stewart's (1970) answer to this question is in the negative, and with this I agree. But from this, I have reached a conclusion opposite to that of Stewart (1970) as to how to use these ideas of splitting and denial.

Stewart (1970) points out that Freud's (1894a) earliest use of this idea of splitting described it as a defense against "incompatible ideas" (p. 47). Stewart further points out that this early idea of splitting is not at all the same as Freud's later use of the concept. First of all, later Freud used this idea of splitting to describe the maintenance of an idea which is in some sense *not-real,* and this is an altogether different matter from the content of one idea simply contradicting or opposing the content of a second idea (see also Segel, 1981). Secondly, splitting later was used by Freud to describe how such a not-real idea is an influence upon the organization of consciousness, and consequently the construction of reality.

A third, and related, source of confusion in Freud's writing about splitting involves the use of this idea by Breuer and Freud (1895d) in their early work on hysteria. Here, recovery into consciousness of defended-against experience was achieved by the use of hypnosis, which brought about an altered state of awareness. An example, noted by Stewart (1970), is how Anna O. was able only via a hypnotic trance to recall a memory of a dog drinking water from a glass.[1] Disgust, embedded in this memory of the dog drinking from the glass, made Anna O. unable to drink liquids. But it is exactly the opposite; *it is the regular presence and consciousness of not-real belief,* which Freud later used so much to describe the operation of splitting and denial. In this investigation I have described the intrinsic relationships which exist among these ideas of playful illusion, splitting, and denial. In papers on the "Infantile Genital Organization," (1923e), the "Economic Problem of Masochism," (1924c), and "Some Psychical Consequences of the Anatomical Distinction between the Sexes" (1945j), Freud repeatedly comes back to the observation about the presence of not-real belief in consciousness. Freud describes how the little boy is conscious about the real absence of a penis in little girls, and, at the same time, maintains in consciousness other beliefs which serve to reassure him: The little boy will also believe that little girls have little penises that cannot be seen, that their penises will soon grow, and so forth. Actually, with splitting (and denial together with playful illusion), certain conscious experiences which may objectively possess contradictory content are not simply subjectively acceptable but are *believed* in some way to be real. It is this characteristic which is emphasized so much in the current concept of splitting. And this is true whether we talk about adult psychopathology or children at an early point in development. Kernberg (e.g., 1966) describes an adult patient "who showed constant switching between severe fears in relation to sexual activities at times and impulse ridden sexual behavior at other times, both alternating conditions being temporarily ego syntonic (p. 236).[1] Kernberg (1966) indicates how such patients would be able to note the appearance of such "severe contradictions in the behavior" (p. 236). But the really important point here is that the content of such contradictory self and/or object representation is experienced with belief when it occurs (Stewart, 1970; Segel, 1981). Kernberg (1966) goes on to say about splitting that it is "alternating expression of complementary sides of a conflict. What are completely separated from each other [and, I would say, equally indexed with belief]. . .are highly complex psychic manifestations, involving affect, ideational content, subjective and behavioral manifestations" (p. 236). Kernberg (1966) concludes that with splitting it is like "two selfs . . . alternating . . . in his conscious experience" (p. 238). Mahler, Pine, and Bergman

(1975), describing children, indicate that with splitting the "mother [representation] is experienced alternately [again with conscious belief] as all good or all bad" (p. 292).

It is important to notice that in the papers written by Freud (1923e, 1924c, 1925j) wherein the little boy is described as maintaining not-real beliefs about anatomical differences, the structural theory (Freud, 1923b) already had been formulated. But notice also that Freud was talking about the maintenance of self and object representations in a pre-Oedipal stage of development, i.e., before the achievement of a mature personality organization differentiated into id, ego, and superego psychic systems. It is with regard to such an immature phase in the life cycle, as Stewart (1970) has stated it, that we can use the idea of a "split" in consciousness because "both the reality and the fantasy coexist" (p. 2). I agree with Stewart that the concept of a split is pertinent to such an early stage in the organization of consciousness and belief. But I suggest a different formulation which derives from the meaning apparatus perspective already described in this investigation. Normal, Oedipal-resolution personality formation into latency includes the emergence of new principles for real to not-real construction, and consequently belief, which in part arise from new capabilities for representation altogether (e.g., Piaget, 1945).

The fantasy versus reality relationship of the older latency child (e.g., Bornstein, 1951) is quite like that of an adult when we compare it to the pre-Oedipal, younger child. The younger, pre-Oedipal child can maintain an organization of consciousness which involves splitting, with belief, because what is subjectively indexed as not-real is play. I already have described how the relationship between play and actuality is entirely different from the later, mature differentiation between fantasy and reality. I also already have stated how I believe that Anna Freud's (1936) contention that the younger child, normally and naturally, possesses a "hypercathexis [of] fantasy" (p. 81) is a congruent statement. But I consider that any such exclusively economic formulation cannot do full justice to the important changes in "thought structures" (Freud, 1900a, p. 542), which are at the heart of the matter. These differences have to do with special characteristics of the immature representational apparatus, which have been illuminated by Piaget (e.g., 1945) and which I have already described.

A final, fourth source of confusion about the idea of splitting in Freud's writing, and something again pointed out by Stewart (1970), involves Freud's (1927e) carrying over this idea to fetishism. The confusion arises from the clinical observation that there is no difference between a fetishist and a psychoneurotic in regard to reality belief, and thus about what is subjectively indexed as real versus non-real in connection with anatomical sex differences. Freud (1927e) always was clear that the construction of the fetishistic object involves a dynamically unconscious fantasy about the existence of a phallic woman. Therefore, fetish construction, Freud stated in the *Outline* (1940a), is like the construction of any neurotic symptom, and this is a "compromise formed with the help of displacement, such as we have been familiar with in dreams" (p. 203). Freud also explicitly stated in the *Outline* (1940a) that it would be "incorrect to describe this process when a fetish is constructed as a splitting of the ego" (p. 203). But if a fetishistic object is so produced by primary processes working upon dynamically unconscious ideas, as is true with any neurotic symptom, then what basis is there to go on to say that the fetishist has a "splitting of the ego" (1940a, p. 203), whereas with the neurotic the not-real belief "is repressed, belongs to the id" (1940a, p. 209)?

Stewart's answer is that there is no basis for such a contention. There is no difference between a fetishistic object and, say, a neurotic phobic object. Both are constructed from a dynamically unconscious idea which has been subjected to primary processes. The fact that one (phobia) attaches anxiety to certain objects and that the other (fetishism) attaches libidinal gratification is clinically important but irrelevant to any idea of splitting. It is interesting to realize that both phobia and fetishistic objects involve a primary process working-over of a *visual* attribute of an object, and this is quite unlike, say, the more strictly ideational symptomatology of the obsessive neurotic. I have suggested elsewhere (Steingart, 1969) that with the advent of post-Oedipal, mature latency personality organization, important individual differences occur with respect to *forms* of organization of consciousness and belief. In particular, a primary emphasis upon imagery may be maintained (versus verbally expressed ideation) although now such imagery essentially is organized according to mature rules of thinking. I suggest that an organization of consciousness which emphasizes imagery is a necessary but obviously insufficient condition for the construction of both phobic and fetishistic objects.[2]

I believe that Stewart's (1970) critical analysis is valuable and correct when he contends that an idea of splitting in mental content is no more relevant to fetishism than it is to neurosis. But I believe that Stewart's (1970) final conclusion based upon this analysis is not productive. Stewart (1970) concludes that we can conceptualize splitting "through various psychopathological levels to the psychotic" (p. 12). Further, Stewart states that there is "no more intimate relationship between the defense of disavowal [denial] and the so-called split in the ego than there is to the defense of repression" (p. 15).

At this point I believe certain observations are in order about Freud's writings on the idea of repression. Freud (1927e) did once use the term denial (disavowal) to designate and differentiate the application of repression to an instinctual idea rather than affective expression. However, in his overall writing, and especially in the *Outline* (1940a), Freud conceptualized an important basis for an important difference between repression and denial (disavowal). Yet, at the same time he did this, he left us with ambiguity about such a difference. Consider this important statement from the *Outline*:

> Let us return to our thesis that the childish ego, under the *domination of the*

> *real world,* gets rid of undesirable instinctual demands by what are called repressions. We will now supplement this by further asserting that, during the same period of life, the ego often enough finds itself in the position of fending off some demand from the external world which it feels distressing and that this is effected by means of a *disavowal* of *the perceptions which bring to knowledge* this demand from reality. Disavowals of this kind occur very often and not only with fetishists; and whenever we are in a position to study them, they turn out to be half-measures, incomplete attempts at detachment from reality. The disavowal is always supplemented by an acknowledgement; two contradictory and independent attitudes always arise and result in the situation of there being a splitting of the ego. (pp. 203–204, first and last italics mine)

There are several points about this citation which are of importance. Freud does not here indicate a framework for a developmental emergence of repression in line with the emergence of the psychic system ego; in fact, Freud here describes repression and denial (disavowal) as events which can occur "during the same period of life" (something emphasized by Segel, 1981). But even here, notice Freud's reference to fetishism and Stewart's (1970) critical analysis, which I have just discussed and with which I agrée. And Freud himself, in other material I just have cited from the *Outline* (1940a, p. 203) appears to realize that it is contradictory to assign fetishistic construction to a concept of splitting, and at the same time say about a fetish that it is produced in the same manner as is a neurotic symptom which is conceptualized to involve repression: This is to say that a fetish construction is a "compromise formed with the help of displacement such as we have been familiar with in dreams" (Freud, 1940a, p. 203). I conclude that we must consider Freud's phrase "during the same period of life" to mean an *entire* period of childhood, pre-Oedipal as well as Oedipal resolution extending into early latency. Denial and splitting pertinent to borderline and narcissistic psychopathology is linked to the former; and repression, connected to neurotic disturbance, is associated with the latter, Oedipal-resolution phase of childhood. In any event, Freud certainly strongly suggests this to be the case in his *Anxiety* monograph (Freud, 1926c), which I will discuss shortly, together with his psychoeconomic viewpoint about these matters. Even here, notice how Freud relates repression versus denial (disavowal) to different *relations to reality* ("domination of the real" versus "incomplete attempts at detachment from reality"). Also, notice the wording, "perceptions which bring to knowledge," involved in Freud's definition of disavowal. What is most important is to realize that in subsequent literature "perception" has become broadened to include *perceptual-like* quality (really everything Freud meant by quality in the Project [1895/1950a]). Thus denial (disavowal) has become implicated and related to affect (e.g., Lewin, 1961) as well as to vivid sensory and motor-filled imagery (e.g., A. Freud, 1936; Jacobson, 1957). But if this be so, and affect as well as such vivid imagery surely relates to instinctual drive expression, then what is the essential difference between denial and repression?

I believe it has to do with what Freud (1940a) touched upon when he spoke about "perceptions which bring to knowledge" (p. 204) some indication of reality. Or this can be put another way, and in a way compatible with the perspective about the development of a meaning apparatus, in terms of how the child develops emerging constructions of knowledge. Denial and repression fundamentally differ with regard to how perception—and now this means any sort of vivid quality—is utilized for the construction of meaning. Denial (disavowal), in part, occurs because an immature psychic apparatus will produce "thought structures" (Freud, 1908, p. 542) which are organized according to some impelling, immediate, perceptual-like quality. Repression (and defenses built upon repression) occurs, in part, because the ideas produced by a more mature psychic apparatus involve meaning structures which possess an autonomy from such immediate, perceptual-like quality. (Actually, in this sense, one can say [e.g., Piaget, 1945] that denial (disavowal) indicates the working of a psychic apparatus which constructs meaning that is *less* detached from a reality known as such only in terms of immediate quality.[3]

Freud (1926d) certainly implies something about the emergent nature of repression in relationship to the development of psychic structure in his *Anxiety* monograph when he states the following:

> It may well be that before its sharp cleavage into an ego and an id, and before the formation of a superego, the mental apparatus makes use of different methods of defense from those which it employs after it has reached these stages of organization. (p. 164)

But interestingly enough, Freud (1915d) is nowhere more explicit about this emergent nature of repression than when he talks in economic terms. Freud's well-known concept, which is the economic counterpart to repression, is, of course, "the assumption of an *anti-cathexis*" (Freud, 1915d, p. 181). Freud (1915d) also significantly added about an anti-cathexis that "It is very possible that it is precisely the cathexis which is *withdrawn* from the idea that is used for anti-cathexis" (p. 181, italics mine). Therefore, this idea of anti-cathexis is not simply a quantitative description of something. It is a *new something*. Anti-cathexis is a construct about an emerging structure—an *anti*-cathexis which is *created* out of another kind of psychic energy. This cathexis which is "withdrawn" is, of course, attention cathexis with which "becoming conscious is connected" (Freud, 1900a, p. 593). It is not, then, as has been suggested, that splitting requires "less counter-cathexis than repression" (Kernberg, 1966, p. 249). I suggest that a formulation in keeping with Freud's ideas would be that splitting involves *no* use of such attention-cathexis-originated counter-cathexis, whereas this emergence of such counter-cathexis is present in the case of repression. There are two further points to be made about this. First, an idea that anti-cathexis is created out of attention cathexis is tantamount to a statement that *systemic* activity is at work—in this case, an ego psychic system. It is, precisely, a defining characteristic of systemic activity that energic interchanges of such a sort can take place (Bertalanffy, 1968). Second, a hypothesis that there now exists repression amounts to a contention that a principle of mental function operates which utilizes psychic tension for further structure formation in the area of defense. The defenses of splitting and denial thus represent in part the pathological counterpart of immature "instinctual vicissitudes" described by Freud (1915c), to which I already have alluded, and none of which involve such counter-cathectic psychic energy.

But neither is it the case that in splitting and denial attention-cathexis is not withdrawn from a conflict provoking instinctual representation. However, with splitting and denial, the attention cathexis which has been withdrawn is not transformed into counter-cathexis. Such withdrawn attention-cathexis is defensively (rigidly and pathologically) applied to another, not-real representation in order to relieve conflict. Jacobson (1957) describes what occurs as follows:

> A general shift of cathexis to the area of perception and apperception, but also a primitive type of perceiving and apperceiving psychic phenomena . . . as if they were concrete parts of the object or of the self. *Withdrawal of cathexis from painful perceptions as well as apperceptions, with simultaneous hyper-cathexis of . . . desirable ones* . . . (p. 126, italics mine)

However, notice that with this term "hyper-cathexis" Jacobson actually does not simply describe the use of a certain kind of psychic energy, but also a *special kind of meaning structure.* While she uses terms like "perceiving and apperceiving," what actually is evident is a special kind of representational structure which organizes meaning in terms of "concrete parts of the object or of the self." I already have suggested that this is nothing else but what Piaget (e.g., 1945) means by preconceptual thought structures, which are symbolized as prototype-images saturated with perceptual-like quality, and now used defensively for the purpose of denial and splitting. Freud (1915e) stated that hyper-cathexis is "no mere act of perception" (p. 194). Indeed it is not. Hyper-cathexis for Freud is the psychic energy counterpart to his theory of meaning. Hyper-cathexes "bring about a *higher psychical organization,*" said Freud, because by such a hyper-cathexis a "thing representation [is] linked with the word-representations corresponding to it" (1915e, p. 202, italics mine).

But here I believe a problem arises in connection with Freud's theory of meaning. Elsewhere (Steingart, 1972) I have stated the opinion that Freud argued too strong a case about the necessity for language acquisition in order for thought to develop into mature, conceptual structures. A young child can be taught to use fairly sophisticated grammatical construction (for example, sentences possessing information about multiple comparisons between two contrasting objects), and conceptual organization still can remain unaffected and immature (Sinclair-deZwart, 1969). Further, research about the cognitive organization of congenitally deaf children, who from birth possess little or no language acquisition, indicates considerable maturity in thought organization (e.g., Furth, 1964; Vernon, 1967; Lennenberg, 1967). I state this again here because there is an important implication in this for the way language may serve (or fool) us in our treatment of young children, or adults who employ the defenses of splitting and denial. I will at least briefly allude to the treatment issue later, but in order to do so, some amplification is required here. The basic point is one already well stated by Wolff (1967). Language is not mechanically (associatively) attached to ideas the way a vineyard label is attached once and for all to a bottle of wine. Here, not only does the wine (thought) mature in the bottle, but also the label (language), and as well the relationship between the two. Therefore, to talk about a cathexis of the "word," (Freud, 1915e, p. 201) which is once and for all attached to a "thing" (Freud, 1915e, p. 201) cathexis, is to leave out of consideration the most important consideration of all, and this is the nature of this attachment, which Piaget (e.g., 1945) refers to as the "symbolic function" (p. 278). Psychoanalysis must work with a theory of cognition which comprehends language and thought as separate phenomena which enter into different relationships with each other at different points in the life cycle. Not surprisingly, it was Hartmann (1953) among psychoanalysts who realized the importance of this signifying function for the development of mature personality organization. Hartmann (1953) stated:

> I would think language, besides adding verbal to thing presentation, is also that function by which the former is made to *signify* the latter (p. 189, italics mine).

But to say that it is "language" which has the "function" to signify is to mix together what actually only is part of the meaning structure—a signifying instrument—with the entire meaning organization which provides meaning. Piaget's work (e.g., 1945) certainly makes clear that, even though the young child may be quite talkative, it is immature preconcepts symbolized as prototype-images which really determine what meanings are comprehended by such language behavior. When this is understood, the way is clear to study how the relationship between language and thought changes with development (see also Vygotsky, 1962). The fact of this changing relationship is significant for the psychoanalytic concept of splitting and denial.

Denial (disavowal) and splitting always implicate a defensive use of preconceptual thought structures for the organization of meaning. Prototype-image representation of a "thing" (Freud, 1915e, p. 201) always is "centered" (Piaget, 1951, p. 235) upon some impelling, perceptual-like quality so that a stable recruitment of meaning is not possible; and belief will be allocated to experience because of insufficient differentiation between representation and actuality (or reality) so represented. Language itself, because it is a socialized, consensually (extrinsically) validated instrument, cannot directly reveal the intrinsic working of such a meaning apparatus. But a proper clinical attention to the language of adults who employ splitting and denial (as well as children) will reveal these characteristics and how they determine meaning. This means that a theoretical differentiation must be made within an overall, general, developmental concept of hyper-cathexis, so that a progressive differentiation and integration of meaning structures can be recognized. One relatively mature kind of hyper-cathexis (organization of meaning) will coincide with the emergence of attention-energy-originated counter-cathectic energy which enables repression.

With this perspective about splitting and denial, it is clear that denial (disavowal) cannot be described as an "intrasystemic mechanism, operating within the ego itself" (Fine, Joseph, and Waldhorn, 1969, p. 53). Denial and splitting do represent procedures for keeping out of awareness the registration of a certain reality or actuality, one which is kept dynamically unconscious. But to conceptualize such a procedure to be an attribute of the theoretical construct psychic system ego is as incorrect as to say that all observation which signals dynamic unconscious activity should be referred theoretically to the construct psychic system id, in disregard of the issue that the id as a psychic system is a product of development (e.g., Schur, 1966). In the same way, we can make observations which obviously have to do with the setting up of ideals, or expectations of punishment over impulses, but these observations need not necessarily be conceptualized to refer to a theoretical construct superego (Hartmann and Lowenstein, 1962). The substantive point is this: Psychoanalysis will make observations that require a conceptualization of psychodynamic conflict over entry into consciousness before the structure, functioning, and content of such conflict *may*develop into an order or organization (differentiation and integration) we then theorize about in terms of (personality mature) id, ego, and superego psychic systems.

Also for these reasons, I do not see how it clarifies matters to suggest that the "concept of denial be reserved for . . . the child's ego . . . matured sufficiently to acknowledge a reality" (Stolorow and Lachmann, 1975, p. 598), or that "splitting, as a defense actively employed by the ego . . . can come into play only after a minimum of integration of oppositely cathected object (and self-)images has been accomplished" (Stolorow and Lachmann, 1978, p. 81) I have emphasized in this investigation that splitting and denial are to be understood as pathological misuses of the way in which the meaning apparatus naturally functions for the young, pre-Oedipal child. But the young pre-Oedipal child has no meaning apparatus capable of any degree of authentic differentiation and integration of experience indexed as real versus not-real, or love versus hate representation. Further, the emergence of the psychic system ego is itself in part determined by the development of such a capability in the meaning apparatus (Steingart, 1969). The problem here is in the failure to recognize that these terms "differentiation" and "integration" represent our most *general* concepts congruent with an equally general idea of development. Indeed, and as I already have stated, the very idea of development itself is inconceivable for psychoanalysis without such concepts of differentiation and integration. But I also have emphasized that psychoanalysis, as a developmental theory, is committed to a position that development over the life cycle always evinces both emerging change and continuity in psychic structure, function, and content. As such, these quite general concepts of differentiation and integration must be understood in themselves to undergo emergent change over the course of the life cycle (Hartmann, 1939). I submit that these ideas of splitting and denial are best understood, and left, to conceptualize a psychopathological misuse of what is already an emergent change in procedures for meaning production which arise with the pre-Oedipal young child.

Here, as always, psychopathology is the master teacher. I take it to be not only an accepted but a required feature of our clinical observation about splitting that an individual who splits mental contents can *remember* that this is what occurs. As Kernberg (1966) puts it, such individuals are "conscious of these severe contradictions in their behavior" (p. 236). But one must emphasize what others (Stewart, 1970; Segel, 1981) already have emphasized, and this is that with splitting a conscious notation of *belief* is attached to each of such "severe contradictions" in experience and behavior. And, while an individual who entertains such belief can be aware in some way that others do not accord his or her illusionary experience a similar status, the individual nevertheless defensively maintains conviction about such not-real experience in the manner of the young child at play.

But there is also another kind of psychopathology about which even such a capability for recollection is absent, and I refer here to a condition variously called "dual personality" (Moore and Fine, 1968, p. 89) or "fugue states" (Moore and Fine, 1968, p. 89) and the like. It cannot serve clarification to apply these concepts of splitting and denial to such a disparate type of psychopathology, for which a term like dissociation is more appropriate. And such qualitative change in psychopathology is not simply a matter of "more" or "less" integration, but the operation of altogether different programs for psychic function and content. Further, if we now view splitting and denial in terms of what will actually occur in later, clinically healthy development, then we also must emphasize another emergent change in psychic structure which produces altogether new types of function and content. All that we need consider is that splitting and denial presuppose a pathological degree of intolerance for different qualities of experience and behavior *which in any event will be recruited to different meanings even for the clinically healthy, pre-Oedipal child.* Such a pathological intolerance already can be observed in a certain kind of disturbed pre-Oedipal child, and such etiology can carry over to an adult in a core area of self and object representation which governs self and object esteem regulation and/or emotional survival. How we can construe a clinically healthy tolerance for such potentially pathological, disruptive experience in early childhood, I will take up in the next section of this investigation.

Also, at least with this viewpoint about splitting and denial, it is clear that to apply in any way the term denial to clinical health (Geleerd, 1965), or to describe splitting as an act of concentration (Stewart, 1970) would only serve to muddy waters. Concentration involves no maintenance in consciousness of split self or object-representation content, or immature belief. Concentration is an adaptive process which is an intentional, *selective* use of available attention cathexes (Rappaport, 1947). Concentration in no way resembles splitting, which is involuntary and mediated outside of awareness, and like any defense shows characteristic pathological rigidity. Also, there is perhaps no great harm done in describing splitting as something "active" (Kernberg, 1975a, p. 25). But activity in the context of splitting means something altogether different from what is meant by activity in the context of adaptation. Actually, if we approach this matter with the useful concepts of activity and passivity supplied by Rappaport (1957a), splitting, like any other inflexible defense against anxiety, is to be understood as passive. Further, I believe the application of the term splitting to "the desired split between observing and experiencing ego in psychoanalysis" (Trunnel and Holt, 1974, p. 272) serves to bring about additional confusion. Self-observation is exactly what people who utilize splitting find so hard to do (e.g., Kernberg, 1975a; Jacobson, 1957; Bach, 1977). Actually, in the experience of self-observation, a person's self representation is an identification which mediates neither the experience of observer nor observee. In self-observation, the person's representation is enabled and mediated by the existence of a structure which interrelates observer and observee experience, and this is a developmental achievement in part made possible by the acquisition of a mature representational apparatus (Steingart, 1969).

Nor do I see how Kohut's (1971) formulation of "a *vertical split in* the psyche in contrast to such *horizontal splits* as those brought about . . . by repression" (p. 177) clarifies matters. First, Kohut seems, in this citation, to equate the idea of a horizontal split with repression. But Kohut (1977) also states the following about "breaking down the barrier that maintained the vertical split" (p. 210):

> The removal of this barrier has the result that the patient will gradually realize that the self-experience in the *horizontally-split* sector of his personality—a self-experience of being empty and deprived which, *although underemphasized, had always been present and conscious*—constitutes his authentic self, and that up till now the predominant self-experience in the non-dichotomized sector—the self experience of overt grandiosity and arrogance—did not emanate from an independent self but from a self that was an appendage to the self of his mother. (p. 210–211, italics mine)

Now Kohut states something different. *Both* pathologically grandiose, arrogant representation, *and* self represenation which possesses qualities of emptiness and deprivation which have been subject to a "horizontal split" *always have had* access to consciousness. Altogether, these concepts of a horizontal and vertical split describe a personality in which grandiose and arrogant self representation is predominant in consciousness; in other words, a quite specific split in mental contents is rigidly maintained at the expense of certain infrequently experienced painful self representation. Inasmuch as we understand repression to mean no access into consciousness whatsoever of the defended against self representation, it is not clarifying to apply the same concept "split" to two such very different circumstances.[4]

Finally, Schafer (1968) offers as an example of splitting an adult who is engaged in a daydream and suggests the following:

> So long as the self is not reflectively represented in relation to the daydream, and is not readily available for such representation . . . [the daydream] may be experienced as real and may therefore gratify to some extent such needs as it expresses. (pp. 92–93)

But I believe even to use the term "daydream" in connection with splitting obscures what is particular and special about splitting and denial, and this has to do with the organization of belief which characterizes consciousness produced by an immature meaning apparatus. Also, Schafer (1968) acknowledges himself that what he terms "reflective self-representations" (p. 92)—thoughts like "I believe" (p. 92) and "It occurs to me" (p. 92)—may also occur during a typical daydream experience. If this be the case, any rationale that the presence or absence of reflective self representation is critical for the maintenance of a daydream versus reality index appears tenuous.

Another comment by Schafer (1968), which is more to the point, is not whether reflective self representation is "readily available," but whether it is "undeveloped" (p. 92). Piaget's work (e.g., 1945) makes clear that, in part, reflective self-observation itself is only one expression of an altogether new organization of meaning which includes an emergent level of differentiation between experience indexed as not-real and as real. In other words, once a mature meaning system is in operation, an index between real and not-real experience is maintained *whether consciously reflected upon or not.* While I have described an important functional difference between childish play and childish illusion, both of these kinds of not-real experience still are to be distinguished from either clinically healthy or neurotic adult experience indexed as not-real, which is a result of such an emergent differentiation in a mature meaning apparatus.

Nevertheless, notwithstanding Freud's (1926b) clear statement about the emergent nature of repression, and thus how repression differs from splitting and denial in a fundamental way, Freud still attempted to use this idea of splitting as an *integrative* concept for all manner of personality (dis)organization and (mal)function. Perhaps the best example of Freud's attempt to use this idea of splitting as such an integrative concept occurs in passages of Lecture Thirty-One of his *New Introductory Lectures* (1933a):

> The ego can take itself as an object, can treat itself like other objects, can observe itself, criticize itself like other objects, can and do Heaven knows what with itself. In this, one part of the ego is setting itself over the rest. So the ego can be split; it splits itself during a number of its functions—*temporarily at least. Its parts can come together again afterwards.* (p. 58, italics mine)

And then Freud quickly goes on to use this idea to illuminate psychopathology with his famous crystal metaphor:

> If we throw a crystal to the floor, it breaks; but not into haphazard pieces. It comes apart along its lines of cleavage into fragments whose boundaries, though they were invisible, were predetermined by the crystal's structure. Mental patients are split and broken structures of this same kind. (p. 59)

But I believe that even here it is clear that the idea of splitting cannot apply to two such very different theoretical contexts. Preyser (1975) already has pointed out how, in the first passage, Freud emphasizes that the "split" is not permanent; Freud (1933a) emphasizes the way "parts come together afterwards" (p. 58). In fact, here Freud is describing *systemic* activity of a coherent personality organization which may or may not be conflicted. In the second paragraph, Freud (1933a) does not use the term ego. Instead, Freud here speaks about "broken structures" (p. 59), which normally would integrate into a coherent organization, and here I believe the idea of splitting and denial properly belong.

Why Freud attempted to use these ideas of splitting and denial in this manner is not difficult to understand. Expressions of Freud's (1895/1950a) original intention in the Project to develop a completely general theory of human behavior and experience persistently surface in his writing, notwithstanding his equally persistent vigilance that he not allow his theory to outrun observation (e.g., Freud 1915e). I consider that Freud believed that in these concepts of splitting and denial he could perform significant integrative work. *His goal, I believe, was nothing less than to use these concepts of splitting and denial to accomplish an integration for vicissitudes of real versus not-real construction as powerful as he had accomplished for sexual behavior with his theory of psycho-sexual drives* (Freud, 1905d). In a paper entitled "The Loss of Reality in Neurosis and Psychosis," Freud (1924e) pointed out that every neurosis "disturbs the patient's relation to reality in some way" (p. 183). Actually, Freud (1911b), in an earlier paper, already had spoken about how "every neurosis has as its result, and probably therefore as its purpose, a forcing of the patient out of real life, an *alienating* of him from reality'' (p. 218, italics mine). This, so-to-speak theoretical ''tilt'' of a neurotic organization of consciousness toward the schizophrenic is complemented by some of Freud's final ideas about splitting in relation to schizophrenia. In the Outline, Freud (1940a) notes that psychotic patients report that, even at the height of their delusional or hallucinatory reconstruction of reality, some veridical reality appraisal remains intact. Freud (1940a) then referred all such phenomena to a concept of a ''psychical split'' (p. 202). Freud then concluded that the idea of splitting is applicable to both neurosis and psychosis, but in the case of neurosis, ''one of these attitudes belongs to the ego and the contrary one, which is repressed, belongs to the id'' (1940a, p. 204). Again we notice what I take to be a theoretically contradictory placement of the concept of splitting in a context of personality development, wherein a coherent psychic system ego is present which utilizes the emergent defense of repression.

But in still another paper, ''Neurosis and Psychosis,'' Freud (1924b) uses an entirely different approach to splitting and denial. Here, I believe, Freud opens the door for us to a quite general comprehension about how not-real experience contributes to personality (dis)organization and (mal) functioning. Furthermore, Freud here portends important contemporary literature, and controversy, about how we are to understand the place of not-real experience in clinical health as well as psychopathology (e.g., Winnicott, 1953; Kohut, 1971; Kernberg, 1974a). Freud in this paper indicated his belief that splitting implicates *neither* neurotic *nor* schizophrenic psychopathology. Splitting here was described as another alternative, which involves what Freud (1924b) called ''encroachments on [psychic] unity'' (p. 152). Freud (1924b) then significantly added the following:

> In this way [i.e., by splitting] the inconsistencies, eccentricities, and follies of men would appear in a *similar light to their sexual perversions*, through the acceptance of which they spare themselves repressions. (p. 153, italics mine)

Freud (1924b) here offers us, through this analogy, ''in a similar light to their sexual perversions'' (p. 153), a profoundly integrative insight about the varieties of not-real to real experience which can occur in clinical health and psychopathology. But we have to imagine for ourselves two different arrays—two triptychs of comparative psychopathology. The first array deals with matters of libidinal and aggressive drive gratification. The second array deals with matters of real to not-real experience and changing psychic structures, function, and content which mediate their interrelationship.

We can place a clinically healthy personality in the center of the first array, with relatively conflict-free, mature psycho-sexual and aggressive forms of drive transformation and development, and this will include a rich amalgam of pre-Oedipal sorts of drive experience as well. On the one side of the center panel in this array, we can place character and symptom neurosis. On the other side we can place fetishism and all perversions which are structured like fetishism. Throughout this entire array it is a mature meaning apparatus, in part, which produces id, ego, and superego psychic systems, together with a structural differentiation between not-real experience as fantasy, and reality. A neurosis can be considered the "negative" (Freud, 1905d, p. 165) of a perversion structured like fetishism, only in the matter of absence or presence of drive gratification. Both the neurosis and fetishism are a result of intersystemic conflict and, accordingly, implicate a complex order of personality differentiation and integration. That there is a background influence of such complex systemic activity is shown in the ego-*alien* quality of the neurotic symptom *and as well* in the uncomfortable "forced" (Fenichel, 1945, p. 324) quality of the fetishistic, perverse experience and behavior.

In the center of the second array, which deals with vicissitudes about the relationship between real and not-real experience, we once again can place a clinically healthy adult personality. The relationship of not-real to real experience for such a person not only is differentiated and integrated by a mature meaning apparatus, but is, as well, relatively conflict-free. I will now adopt and reverse a term coined by Winnicott (1953), "imaginative living" (p. 14), to describe such a state of affairs. The developmental, functional (but not structural) ancestor of such "imaginative living" is what I have described already, the play of the clinically healthy young child. Loewald (1975) has given a recent emphasis to the need for a revised view of this relationship between not-real imagination and experience indexed as real, in a clinically healthy adult personality:

> But a fantasy is unreal only insofar as its communication with present actuality is inhibited or severed. . . . Perhaps a better word than "unreal" is "meaninglessness." (p. 289)

and

> In the healthier adult, communication and interplay between the world of fantasy and the world of objectivity, between imagination and rationality, remain alive. (p. 290)

On the one side of the center panel in this array we place *both* neurosis and fetishism (and all perversion structured like fetishism). All such psychopathology exhibits what Freud (1911b) termed "fantasy which is alienating [i.e., conflicted] from reality" (p. 218). But the psychopathology which occupies the third and last panel of this second array goes beyond conflict which is nevertheless still experienced within a matrix of firm differentiation between not-real and real experience. Here we locate what I have already described as playful illusion, which is a "positive" expression of what I have called a meaning disturbance (splitting and denial). Such psychopathology represents a direct continuation of functional psychopathology in the young child which produces pathological illusion rather than healthy play.

Notice that throughout the description of these two arrays of adult, comparative psychopathology, I have not used the diagnostic term schizophrenia. I believe it is correct not to do so. The essential manifest feature of schizophrenia obviously is not some matter related to drive development and gratification. Nor is schizophrenic delusional or hallucinatory reconstruction of reality (or language and thought disorder) the same as what I have described as a meaning disorder, as playful illusion. But with respect to such playful illusion, I am now in the position to take advantage of the important analogy hinted at by Freud (1924b): *Pathologically playful illusion is a kind of "perversion" with regard to the relationship between real and not-real experience, such as that which perverse experience and behavior accomplishes in the area of drive gratification.*

With this behind me, I now can turn my attention to a large area of relatively recent literature which deals with adult conditions variously termed borderline, narcissistic, false-self, schizoid, psychotic-character, and so forth, psychopathology (e.g., Kernberg, 1975a; Kohut, 1971; Bach, 1977; Deutsch,1942; Frosch, 1970; Winnicott, 1968). The diagnostic question for this entire area of psychopathology—an intermediate area which intuitively impresses us as neither neurotic nor schizophrenic—is the same as would be the differential assessment question for any major diagnostic category: What is the essential and regular feature of this third kind of psychopathology? I am now in a position to say that what characterizes this entire, distinct third region of psychopathology is the maintenance of what I have called a meaning disturbance as pathological play in a core area of representation which governs self/object esteem and/or emotional survival.

Moreover, I believe it is the *capacity* of some such individuals not just to emphasize, but to make critically but rigidly important for themselves a treatment relationship based upon gratifying, grandiose, and idealizing playful illusion enabled by such a meaning disturbance, which constitutes our psychoanalytic yardstick for the presence of narcissistic personality psychopathology.[5] I also suggest that when such a meaning disturbance especially, or in alternating fashion, produces psychically painful mental content—and especially experience infiltrated with orally based aggression projected and otherwise (Kernberg, e.g., 1975a)—we tend toward a diagnosis of borderline personality. This also can be understood as pathological play, but now pathological play which is psychically painful rather than gratifying. It is altogether different in function from fluid, expected episodes of frightening play produced by a clinically healthy child which is in the service of mastery and adaptation.

I am, of course, mindful of literature about such narcissistic or borderline, etc., individuals which conceptualizes such psychopathology in terms of separation-individuation disturbance (e.g., Mahler and Kaplan, 1977; Settledge, 1977; Pine, 1979); and it is not that I disagree with any contention that such disturbance is regularly present. But I do maintain that what strikes the clinician more immediately is this matter of a not-real (but not schizophrenic) transference relationship. Further, there is another type of psychopathology—predominating addictive states which involve alcohol, drugs, food, sexuality, etc.—and about such individuals we also believe separation-individuation disturbance to be critical. I do not believe that individuals who present with such a predominating addictive state empathically impress us to be people who can maintain such a not-real (but not schizophrenic) transference relationship; indeed, I believe that the addictive state of consciousness defensively stands in the place of this. Certainly we are familiar with the difficulty of maintaining a viable treatment relationship with such addictive individuals. One can begin to think, about addictive-state individuals, that their separation-individuation disturbance derives from an earlier "practicing" (e.g., Mahler, Pine, and Bergman, 1975, p. 291) phase, and contrast this with "rapprochement" (Mahler, Pine, and Bergman, 1975, pp. 291–292) psychopathology which enables a playful illusionary transference relationship, but I suspect that this approach is too simple.

Thus, I repeat that the essential and regular feature of this entire intermediate area of adult psychopathology is what I have called and described as a meaning disturbance (which already can be observed in a certain kind of disturbed young child). It occurs because such adults continue a pathological misuse of an immature "symbolic function" (Piaget, 1945, p. 278) in a core area of self and object representation. I also repeat the important consequence of this for psychopathology: (1) Prototype, vivid sorts of perceptual, kinesthetic, etc., experience enter into self and object representation, and such representations operate like immature "pre-concepts" (Piaget, 1945, p. 221). Therefore, self and object representation which may possess unrealizable but impelling grandiose, idealizing, destructive, etc., content will continue a "participation" (Piaget, 1945, p. 226) in the existence of some actuality or reality. The "positively" felt result of this is playful illusionary belief. (2) Inasmuch as mature conceptual structure for self and object representation does not exist, discrete, actually unique and individual referents (inanimate things, persons, relations) are not known as such; each will "participate" (Piaget, 1945, p. 228) directly with each other, and so lose stable mental content. This only says the same thing in two different ways: Only if the symbolic representation is fully differentiated can it function for an individual to secure stable reference (meaning) for referents relevant to self and object representation; only with authentic self and object representation can linguistic and other symbols which signify such representation be differentiated from something now known to be reality (referents). But certainly it is clinically important to understand not only what is regular but also what is varied about this nonneurotic and nonschizophrenic third area of adult psychopathology.

What appears to be variable are the particular kinds of mental contents repetitively used for denial and splitting as well as how rigidly maintained is such split and denied mental content.

Certainly, in the literature on narcissistic personalities, what is emphasized is the repetitive and rigid maintenance of pathological grandiose and/or idealized content which directly relates to self and object esteem (e.g., Kohut, 1971, 1977; Kernberg, 1975; Bach, 1977). I have described how the application of Piaget's idea of immature, preconceptual meaning structure, carried over to social experience, is Piaget's corollary (e.g., 1945) concept of egocentrism. This idea of a pathological, rigid maintenance of such egocentrism has been used by Bach (1977) to comprehend how narcissistic personalities do not possess what he terms a "reflective self" (p. 211). The presence of such a self representation would be signaled by the psychic function of self-observation. I have indicated how self-observation implicates an identification structure which is neither only the perspective of one person, or the other, but is a structured relationship of two or more people now known to be in an interaction. Bach (1977) also applied this Piagetian perspective to other features of adult narcissistic personality reported in the literature, such as absence of any experience of self-initiative, or identity continuity, and egocentric use of language, as well as extreme mood swings (with regard to identity continuity and mood swings also see Steingart [1969]). But these sorts of features—an inability to maintain the reality of plural perspectives, lack of stable identity content, lack of a sense of initiative, egocentric language, extreme mood swings—appear to characterize this entire group of nonneurotic and nonschizophrenic psychopathology. Deutsch (1942), over thirty-five years ago, described what has come to be called an "as if" personality, who shows a continuous, *unknowing* (i.e., egocentric) replacement of self representation in an imitation of each new love object. Now such adult psychopathology might be referred to the more recent concept of an *idealized* self-object (Kohut, 1971). But the point here is that Deutsch did not herself emphasize the self-esteem aspect of such a state of affairs, but instead chose to emphasize the inability to maintain an object relationship in any way other than through such a total, imitative-identification. Kernberg's (e.g., 1975a) description of borderline personality appears to emphasize splitting which is more directly related to matters of hateful representation, although he certainly does not leave out splits in mental content which bear more directly upon self-esteem. Kernberg (1975a) also emphasizes that more "integrated" (p. 265) functioning is found to exist in certain narcissistic personalities compared to borderline individuals. But I suspect that we deal with a matter of relative rigidity in split mental contents rather than any sort of authentic integration. Further, I believe Winnicott (1968) would consider any such appearance of integration to be a feature of a "compliant false self" (p. 146) personality organization, and all together, he describes a kind of individual whose splits in mental content can be quite subtle with respect to ordinary observation. It is, of course, of interest and importance to understand the differential etiologies of all of these different sorts of meaning disturbance. While I am convinced that, at least to some extent, real differences of these sorts do exist, there is also a question of the extent to which differences in clinical practice and conceptual orientation produce this variety. However this may be, I come back to my point that the essential, regular feature of all such adult psychopathology is what I have called a meaning disturbance: This is a misuse of cognition for pathological play which will be gratifying or painful.[6]

I also believe that this perspective argues for a change in the fulcrum of discussion with respect to the Kernberg-Kohut controversy (e.g., Kernberg, 1974b; Ornstein, 1974; Kernberg, 1975b) about our theory of narcissistic personality disorder. The question is not whether the grandiose and idealized representations of the clinically healthy young child are as thoroughly unrealizable as those of the adult individual with a narcissistic personality disturbance—they are essentially the same in this respect—and here I believe I express my agreement with Kohut (1971). But neither can one conclude from this that adult narcissistic disturbance is a simple arrest of childhood grandiosity and idealization. I believe Kernberg (1975a) is correct when he states that the clinically healthy "child's. . .need to be the center of attention, admiration, and love, *coexists* with simultaneous expression of genuine love. . .in his objects" (p. 272, italics mine). Further, I believe that what Kohut (e.g., 1971) describes as a normal "transmuting internalization [of self regard]" (p. 50) will be determined in part precisely by whether or not there is present such genuine object love as well as narcissistic involvement.[7] I do not believe one can create such clinically healthy psychic structure *only* out of even benevolent projective identifications. I also agree with Kernberg (1975a) that the "grandiose [and I will add idealized] fantasies of normal, small children. . . have by far a more realistic quality than is the case of narcissistic personalities" (p. 272). But I mean by this not the contents of such representations in themselves but *the presence of a flexible, easy relationship in the clinically healthy young child between such grandiose and idealized content about self and object representations and other representations which are produced by such changing actualities as hunger, fear, death of a parent, etc., in the child's life.* In other words, what is central is whether such childish grandiosity and idealization remain like healthy play or become what I have called playful illusion. The next question then becomes what determines this defensive movement of normal, childish grandiose or idealized play into defensive illusion. Here again I think what is needed is a somewhat changed perspective. My experience is in agreement with Kernberg (e.g., 1975a). Orally based envy and aggression provoke such defensive movement of play into illusion. But another important *determinant* of what makes for such rage and envy, which in turn fosters pathological illusion, is exactly some disturbed response on the mother's part to her child's normal and natural playful grandiosity and idealization. Here I think that Kohut (e.g., 1971) makes an important contribution to our theory and practice.

But to recognize such a mutually constitutive, reciprocal relationship between narcissistic and object-invested drive pleasures hardly calls for some theoretical "independent line of narcissistic development" (1971, p. 6). For Freudian psychoanalysis such clinically healthy grandiosity and idealization always will enter into a mutually constitutive relationship with object-invested instinctual drive experience. Actually, Kohut (1977) himself eloquently describes this complex array:

> If a mother accepts the fecal gift proudly—or if she rejects it or is uninterested in it—she is not only responding to the drive. She is also responding to the child's forming self. Her attitude, in other words, influences the set of inner experiences that play a crucial role in the child's further development. She responds—accepting, rejecting, disregarding—to a self that, in giving and offering, seeks confirmation by the mirroring self-object. (pp. 75-76)

Certainly we can conceptualize different aspects of this whole experience, and so differentiate drive-related experience from narcissistic pleasures, among others. These different aspects will indeed call for differential therapeutic interpretation with different people, at different times in the treatment relationship. But I believe that Kohut's (e.g., 1971, 1977) argument for a theoretically separate psychology of the self is itself a theoretical mirroring which does not affirm the nature of the actual, complex psychic reality. Furthermore, I believe that in this very example I have cited Kohut works against the point he wants to make. It is not simply that the mother accepts the fecal gift "proudly" (i.e., narcissistically gratifyingly), which secures the child's development into individuated self-esteem regulation. I believe, for example, that clinical experience with certain obsessive neurotic psychopathology indicates that a mother may characteristically respond with a disturbed disgust over the same fecal gift, and yet development into individuated self-esteem regulation will go forward. The point here is that there are other, vital matters about this mother-child relationship which will determine whether the young child will experience the meaning of the fecal product as something created by himself or herself. These matters have to do with the relationship of real to not-real experience in the development of love, hate, and ambivalence, to which I now turn.

6

On Real and Not-Real Meaning in Love, Hate, and Ambivalence

I want now to consider how a certain development in procedures for meaning production in the young pre-Oedipal child, especially with regard to not-real experience, is a necessary but insufficient condition for the emergence of love, hate, and ambivalence. What is most pertinent is how an understanding about the development of certain procedures for meaning production enables one to have a better understanding of self-enhancing omnipotence or grandiosity as well as object-enhancing idealization. Omnipotence (grandiosity), together with idealization, always has been considered to be intimately related to love experience. With this accomplished, I will develop congruent ideas for hate experience as well as ambivalence. Finally, in connection with ambivalence, I take up the concept of self and object representational constancy and consider what meaning this can have in early childhood.

I will speak about the *developmental achievement* of love, hate, and ambivalence. I want to work out the contribution made by the meaning apparatus to such a developmental accomplishment. I believe this has to do with an interplay of not-real experience to reality (or actuality in the young child), and that the route to such an understanding of this is by way of Freud's (1914c) concepts of omnipotence and idealization. With these concepts of omnipotence and idealization, I surely am in the territory of not-real experience. But how, exactly, is love to be understood as not-real experience? And what is the relevance of the features of a person's meaning apparatus to the development of self-enhancement omnipotence and object-enhancement idealization which we consider intrinsic to love (Freud, 1914c)? And further, when does love begin in the life cycle? I will begin with the last question and speak about the *emergence of love* in early childhood. I also will go on to maintain that when love begins, there also emerge other, new, probably distinctively human experiences for which the terms hate and ambivalence should be reserved.

We have come, in our theory, to the important realization that neither the instinctual drives nor objects are to be considered as simply given as *psychic* phenomena (e.g., Jacobson, 1964; Schur, 1966; and more recently, see especially Loewald, 1971). A species-specific (human) organismic potential for the production of meaning enters into a mutually constitutive relationship with environmental sources to produce, altogether, psychic instinctual drive, together with self and object *representation.* Whatever other useful sociological or interpersonal frameworks can be applied to these concepts of self and object representation (e.g., Mead, 1934; Sullivan, 1940; Goffman, 1959), for Freudian psychoanalysis self and object representation originate and always remain rooted in instinctual drive notation. But all of this has to do with the organism-environment encounter involved in the *origin* of human motivation, instinctual and aggressive *drive* representation, and not with a later acquisition of what I will call the bio-social desires of love and hate. An initial, mutually constitutive relationship between human organism and environment creates a representational world: instinctual drives which show a "fitting together" (Hartmann, 1939, p. 38) with distinct but extensive oral, anal, etc., self and object schemata (see, for example, Wolf, 1967; Schimeck, 1975). I here allude to the valuable formulation made by Hartmann. Hartmann (1939) describes a "*reality principle in the broader . . . sense*" (p. 44); this reality principle "can even regulate the possibilities of pleasure gain" (p. 44) in the service of Homo sapiens species adaptation. There is nothing particularly complicated or mysterious about this. For example, Homo sapiens has evolved such that it is psychically pleasurable for each individual human baby to eat food which is brought into contact with the mouth. And the variety of foods which can thus take on an eventual psychic representation of oral pleasure is broad so that human species survival is facilitated. From this point of view, we can understand Freud's (1915c) statement that the object "is what is most variable about an instinct" (p. 122).

But it is altogether different with love and hate. Once libidinal instinctual gratifications have become involved with a love object, so long as love is maintained, this object of libidinal gratification is the *least variable thing about an instinct.* Also, once libidinal gratifications have become involved with a love object, anxiety which formerly only had to do with an absence of gratification (object loss) *now also inheres in the gratification experience itself.* I now will elaborate upon these two matters.

Freud (1914c) once described love objects as "those which satisfy the needs of *sublimated* sexual instincts" (p. 137, italics mine). And about idealization versus sublimation, Freud (1914c) said this:

> Sublimation . . . consists in the instinct's directing itself toward an aim otherthan, and remote from that of sexual satisfaction; in this process the accent falls upon *deflection* from sexuality. . .Insofar as sublimation describes something that has to do with instinct and idealization something to do with the object, the two concepts are to be distinguished from each other. (p. 94, italics mine)

But how can such an idea of sublimation—a concept that involves a remoteness from libidinal gratification—be related to love? Certainly with clinically healthy love, whether we consider its inception in young children or adults, we expect a certain consummation of libidinal gratification rather than any sort of deflection of libidinal aim. We can, in a special way, keep the essence of some such idea of a "deflection" of libidinal gratification in love. But we must understand that the "deflection" of libidinal gratification which occurs in love is not *away* from a sexual aim. Quite the opposite, what transpires in love is that the libidinal gratification is deflected, one might say, "upward" into what I will call an *exaltation*, a not-real stratification of the gratification experience itself. This exaltation of the libidinal drive experience itself, in love, is directly and especially experienced as *romance.* It is this emergence of a now transformed libidinal gratification into romance which also shows a natural "fitting together" (Hartmann, 1939, p. 38) with an idealized (particular, special) love object.

And about idealization, when can we say we first observe it in the life cycle? I take the position that we first—but not quite—observe idealization with the advent of the transitional object. Winnicott (1953) states that transitional object phenomena "begins to show" (p. 4) when an infant is anywhere from four to twelve months of age. But we know that idealization—taken now as a special quality which attaches to the *representation* of a love object—ordinarily cannot occur until around the end of the first year, or often between a year and eighteen months, because representation altogether only emerges at such a time (see, for example, Piaget, 1952; Fraiberg, 1969; Bell 1970). I agree here with Metcalf and Spitz (1978), who indicate that the "period of the transitional object and its vicissitudes has not as yet been sufficiently investigated" (p. 104). But the substantive point is that it is an essential vicissitude of the transitional object *to develop.* The transitional object develops in this way: At first, the transitional object is a concrete thing only *associated* with a mother who is not yet psychically represented as physically individuated, and hence only is "known" by her child to be in perfect, sensory-motor, symbiotic fusion. Then the transitional object becomes a vehicle, a "symbolic function" (Piaget, 1951, p. 278) which now *represents* such a not-real perfect state versus the representation of the actualities of mother-child physical individuation. It is only with the latter, and later, emergence that we can speak about the "magic *evocative* power" of the transitional object, or how this object can come to represent a perfect, symbiotic "golden age" (Metcalf and Spitz, 1978, p. 105, italics mine). Then, for example, a symbolic function expressed in the transitional object will enable the fretful child to go to sleep (see Fraiberg's [1969] comments about evocative memory; and see also Passman and Weisberg [1975] for a discussion of experimental literature which is congruent with such a developmental viewpoint).[1]

At another time, Freud (1933a) connected love with instinctual gratifications that are "inhibited in their aim . . . so that a *lasting* object cathexis comes about. Such, for instance, is the relation of *tenderness* . . . " (p. 97, italics mine). This idea of Freud's, that with love there emerges a "tenderness" which is "lasting," is congruent with Bergmann's (1980) recent emphasis upon the experience of longing and his idea that "longing. . .marks the birth of love" (p. 72). But again, I believe it runs counter to our actual experience with clinically healthy love to believe that tenderness or longing is produced by any sort of inhibition of sexual desire. The experience of tenderness or longing, I suggest, has to do with earlier, pre-Oedipal sources of libidinal gratification, especially oral, which normally become involved in clinically healthy love and participate in this general not-real exaltation of the gratification experience. We owe to Freud (1905d) himself the insight that adult human sexuality is a complex pulling-together of diverse sources of libidinal gratification; and, I add, the not-real exaltation of libidinal drive experience, together with self and object representation, which is intrinsic to clinically healthy love, will of necessity also express such a variated source.

I therefore conclude that neither of these unique characteristics of love—its "lasting . . . tenderness" (Freud, 1933a, p. 97) or its romance—can be described, let alone explained, with concepts such as inhibition or sublimation, which only modify what still remains an idea of an *untransformed* libidinal drive. Rather, with love, there occurs (along with object representation idealization) a transformation into exaltation of the representation of the libidinal drive gratification itself. One can state this from a viewpoint of psychic energy, economically, and say the following: The sexual instinct now has changed from a preemptory but periodic drive (Rappaport, 1960) to a bio-social *desire* which is relatively *continuously* in need of fulfillment. Speaking now from the viewpoint of a young childwho operates with an immature meaning apparatus, love is an emergent type of desire quality which will center about new prototype images of the mother herself (e.g., her hair), and this is altogether different from any sort of representation centered about some vicissitude of libidinal drive gratification (e.g., sucking, biting, etc.).

But the emergence of love not only involves not-real exaltation of the drive experience representation (romance and tenderness) together with idealization of the love object. Love also involves what Freud called (1914c) omnipotence for the self representation, or to use Kohut's (e.g., 1971) more contemporary term, grandiosity. In order to explicate this, I now want to make plain that this description of love is also my interpretation of certain comments made by Winnicott (1954a) about what he called a "*new* kind of need [which] has arisen based on impulse. . . . Risk has entered in" (p. 267, italics mine). And it is now time to cite some relevant passages from Winnicott's (1954a) writing about the "high order of complexity" (p. 263) which characterizes the emergence of love in the young child's relationship to the mother. Even what follows is not a full description of this complexity.

> In simplest possible terms the excited baby . . . becomes carried away by crude instinct and with *ideas* of the powerful kind that belong to instinct. (We must assume a relatively satisfactory feed, or other instinctual experience.) (p. 267, italics mine)

> Some anger at frustration is of course part and parcel even of satisfactory feeding. (p. 269)
>
> The mother is not the same after as before. . . . what the infant feels [is that] there is a hole, where previously there was a full body of richness. (p. 268) For our purposes here, this infant, after the feed . . . [is] apprehensive about the imagined hole in the body of the mother [and] is also very much caught up in the struggle within the self, struggle between what is felt to be good . . . and what is felt to be bad. . . . (p. 269)
>
> The infant that is blessed with a mother who survives, who knows a gift gesture when it is made, is now in a position to do something about that hole. . . made in the original instinctual moment. Here come in the words reparation and restitution. . . . The *gift gesture may reach to the hole*, if the mother plays her part. . . . *The healthy child has a personal source of sense of guilt*, and need not be taught to feel guilty or concerned. (p. 270, first italics mine)
>
> For a long while the small child needs someone who is not only loved but who will *accept potency . . . in terms of reparative and restitutive giving*. . . . It is a sure sign of a lack of understanding of small children . . . when an adult thinks to help by giving, failing to see the primary importance of being there *to receive*. (p. 271, italics mine)

There are a number of matters which are of great importance in these comments by Winnicott.

It is instructive to compare these comments by Winnicott with the teaching by Jesus that "It is more blessed to give than to receive" (Acts 20:34). What Winnicott here is telling us is that, with clinically healthy love, the lover is not more but equally as blessed as the beloved. I take it to be self-evident that clinically healthy love experience always involves a simultaneous not-real elevation for both self and object representation. Now it is, of course, well known that Freud (1914c) worked with a model of a finite amount of psychic energy which could lead him to say that "broadly speaking an antithesis" (p. 76) exists as regards the investment of libidinal psychic energy into either self or object representation. However, even within such a theoretical context, it is the term "broadly" which should be emphasized. Therefore, it does not necessarily follow, as has been suggested (Fromm, 1956), that even such a finite psychic energy model would lead to an expectation that a lover must experience him or herself as empty or depleted compared to an idealized, beloved other. Freud (1914c) did say, "A strong egoism is a protection against falling ill" (p. 85), but he also said, "Men are bound to fall ill if, in consequence of frustration, we are unable to love" (p. 85). Jacobson (1953b) has emphasized how "normal functioning . . . presupposes a sufficient and *evenly* distributed libidinous cathexis of both the object and self-representation" (p. 60, italics mine), and I will speak more about this shortly. But now there is still this vital characteristic of love which has to do with a stratification of experience into not-real self-representation grandiosity and object-representation idealization. Theoretical parameters about locale and amount of libidinal investment cannot explicate clinically healthy or pathological vicissitudes which have to do with a stratification of experience into experience which is in some way indexed as real or actual versus not-real. Consider, for example, some psychopathology: We consider that both pathological paranoid grandiosity and obesity indicate a similar unhealthy over-investment of libidinal drive in self representation. But only in the former do we have schizophrenic, not-real experience, whereas in the latter what is present is only an extremely large physical body.

These comments by Winnicott (1954a), which I have taken to be theory about the emergence of love, do help us understand how it is that not-real experience inheres in love, and how the young child's meaning apparatus contributes to this "new kind of need" (p. 267). The young child egocentrically knows and feels that a new play-like idealized mother experiences herself as emptied out of something good as a consequence of the libidinal gratification the mother has provided. This produces a natural concern in the young child to replenish the mother. And, again egocentrically, the young child knows and feels that the now idealized mother experiences herself as restored by virtue of the libidinal gratification the child provides to the mother. The restoration or replenishment effected by the young child naturally substantiates the child's self representation as a good someone who can be a potent, clinically healthy, play-like, grandiose provider of *happiness*, which now includes, but is more than, relatively simple straightforward gratification. The realization by the child of this clinically healthy not-real experience—that what he or she provides the mother is not ordinary but an extraordinary "gift gesture" (Winnicott, 1954a, p. 270)—is the root of the inherent emotional tally between narcissistic satisfaction and love. Therefore, one can realize that narcissism is not related directly to libidinal gratification but to love which develops out of such gratification. Thus, the young child unknowingly (i.e., egocentrically) replenishes the idealized mother representation as a future source of happiness-producing libidinal gratification for himself or herself by virtue of the mother's being made happy by the child.

If I go back to some of my earlier, general comments about development, I can also take these comments by Winnicott to mean the following: A life instinct principle of mental function, which utilizes psychic tension to produce emergent structure, now has operated in the area of motivation. The young child now has developed from a relatively simple straightforward matter of libidinal gratification via an object to a more complex psychic organization, which I will call the *fulfillment of love desire*. The young child now is making love.

Notwithstanding the young child's egocentric and primitive comprehension of what transpires in love, indeed in order to enable this natural operation of an immature meaning apparatus with the emergency of love, the following *actual* conditions must be supplied by the mother. The mother must be able emotionally to survive being "attacked" (Winnicott, 1954a, p. 266) by her child's love desire together with any degree of hatred based upon imperfectly felt fulfillment. Emotional survival means no inappropriately excessive emotional withdrawal, depression, anger of her own, or whatever. That is, the young child must be able to elicit a vivid (good enough) demonstration on the mother's part that emotionally she "continues to exist" (Winnicott, 1948, p. 161) during his or her gratification experience. Also, and just as important, the mother must show a vivid (good enough) demonstration that she can be happily pleasured by the child; that is, that the young child's "gift gesture" (Winnicott, 1954a, p. 270) has an *effect*.

Also, I once again come back to the meaning apparatus perspective and emphasize some things Winnicott takes for granted. The young child, with the emergence of love, thinks, has representation of, for example, a hole, of himself or herself, as well as the mother. And the young child, with love, knows and feels a self representation which is now in a fundamental, *physical way* individuated from the mother representation. A term, for example, like reparation makes sense only if we presuppose such a knowing by the child about the physical existence of two individuated, physical beings. Also, I want to tie in here my earlier comments about the advent of the transitional object. The initial occurrence of the transitional object implicates not only the soon-to-emerge representational capabilities, but also a not-real versus actual stratification of meaning about experience to be so represented. In other words, with the emergence of love-making, the young child possesses and uses meanings which pertain to an idealized (or degraded) versus actual mother, as well as a grandiose (or humiliated) versus actual self.

One cannot say about relatively healthy love that it is either passive or active. Altogether, the entire experience can be understood to be fashioned after the sheer physical eroticism between two people which is such a vital ingredient in romantic love. When a lover touches or strokes the beloved, he or she is, at the same time, the agent of pleasure as well as the recipient.

Nor should one say about clinically healthy love that it is a choice, or better stated, a kind of forced choice between experience in some way indexed as real or actual and not-real enhancement of self and other. Freud (1914c) once described something he called a "narcissistic type" (p. 90) of object involvement, by which he meant an attachment to another which is replete with not-real enhancement for self and object representation. I believe it is Kohut's (e.g., 1971) important contribution to emphasize, with his concept of a "self-object" (p. 90), how it is a natural, psychological process for the young child to understand and feel, say, self-grandiosity or object idealization to be a matter of a positive resonance between a parent and a child who are treated with respect to esteem regulation as one and the same individual. But Freud (1914c) also described for the young child what he called an "anaclitic" (p. 90) attachment. I understand this to mean another sort of relationship founded upon another psychological actuality possessed by this same young child. And this is that, indeed, he or she and the parents have, in fact, two separate and very different individual bodies, from which derives a fundamental actuality that parents provide for the child in all manner of ways because the child cannot provide for himself or herself. In fact, Freud (1914c) emphasized such actualities in his descriptions of "anaclitic" (p. 90) attachment as "the woman who feeds [and] the man who protects" (p. 90). I consider that the emergence of clinically healthy love is built upon both narcissistic and anaclitic sorts of object involvement. The former emphasizes not-real grandiose and idealized mental contents, whereas the latter emphasizes mental contents which relate to the actualities which exist between young child and parents. It is the latter, actuality-centered mental content which enables one to say that a clinically healthy young child's love includes authentic—that is, non-narcissistic—investment and interest in the existence of the other as a separate person. The young child's capacity for this actuality-centered relationship is something emphasized by Kernberg (1975a), with which I agree; and it is a point still more recently emphasized by Gediman (1975), Bergmann (1980), and Kaplan (1978). And I repeat: It is precisely characteristic of clinically healthy love, for both young child and adult, that it is a relatively smooth, functional integration of such diverse but potentially conflictual or disorganizing experiences. Indeed, I add a stress that love must involve both not-real, narcissistic, and actuality-centered, anaclitic attachments if it is to have a chance to be clinically healthy. I stress the term "functional" because, for the young child, a meaning apparatus does not yet exist which can actually organize such qualitatively diverse experience into a coherent meaning structure (Piaget, e.g., 1951). Nevertheless, just as I have described in general regarding play versus actuality, a similar free and easy interplay is to be expected between narcissistic and anaclitic object attachment aspects of a love relationship for the young child. It is a conflict-instigated overemphasis of *either* the not-real, narcissistic, or actuality-centered, anaclitic attachment aspects of love which signals an emotional disturbance in the young child (or adult). This constitutes another argument against a theoretical conception that narcissism follows an "independent" (Kohut, e.g., 1971, p. 6) line of development. But it remains true that it is the narcissistic (idealized-grandiose) aspect which carries the not-real spark which can make of love such an electric experience throughout life.

With regard to this narcissistic aspect of love in early childhood, a state of affairs is now present in which self and object esteem regulation extends in a unitary manner over two individuals who are actually (objectively) separate. I have said it is Kohut's (e.g., 1971, 1977) important contribution to emphasize the naturalness of this kind of esteem regulation structure early in the life cycle, and one which is congruent with the normalcy of cognitive egocentricism also characteristic of the young child. But the normalcy of such cognitive egocentrism and "self-object" (Kohut, e.g., 1971, p. 90) esteem regulation at this point in the life cycle ought not to obscure the fact that the young child can—indeed must—experience him or herself as a separate someone who can *make love* occur in order for clinically healthy development to take place. Notwithstanding the fact that esteem regulation is not individuated, some degree of authentically individuated object investment is present with the young child (Kernberg, 1975a; Bergmann, 1980; Kaplan 1978). But how are we to conceive of what enables (mediates) this possibility? While esteem regulation is not yet completely individuated between parent and child, their two separate physical bodies are known and felt as such by the young child. I believe this vital competence to make love especially is mediated by the physical eroticism which is so natural to this period (hugging, kissing, etc.). It is this vital competence to make love which is one important basis of what Kohut (1977) describes as a "nuclear self" and an "independent center of initiative" (p. 177).

I now can make a complete statement about the phenomenology of this fulfillment of love desire: There is a natural "fitting together" (Hartmann 1939, p. 38) of romance and tenderness (via libidinal drive exaltation), with an elevated love object (via idealization), together with an enhanced self-representation (via omnipotence, or to use Kohut's [1971] more contemporary term, grandiosity).[2] I emphasize Hartmann's (1939) terms "fitting together" (p. 38) deliberately because I believe this entire, emerging complex of love also possessed and possesses individual and species survival value. Our primitive ancestors, after all, were not especially strong or swift compared to a large number of other land animals, especially so in prehistoric times, and they could not fly to escape land predators. It always has been extraordinarily rare for the human female to produce a litter, and the single infant at a time characterizes the species. There probably never was a biologically "guaranteed" mating time or season in Homo sapiens to the extent that this exists elsewhere in nature, which apparently makes us unique among life forms (Udry and Morris, 1968). But in place of a guaranteed mating time or season, we have love desire which is relatively continuously in need of fulfillment, and this certainly must have supported reproduction of the species. Just as important, love desire promoted that kind of intense bonding which facilitated close familial (herd) ties which provided safety in prehistoric times. What I am at least suggesting is that, over the long evolutionary haul, Homo sapiens species survival and individual selection was as much an affair of the heart as the activity of the mind, and probably in some manner the two mutually constituted each other.[3] This last idea is not original with me. Freud (1915b) certainly expressed comments which are similar when he stated the following:

> What released the spirit of inquiry in man was not the intellectual enigma [of death], and not every death, but the *conflict* of feeling at the death of *loved* yet alien and hated persons. Of this conflict of feeling psychology was the first offspring. (pp. 293–294, italics mine)

At still other times, Freud (1912d) described love as including, in addition to the sensual, an "affectionate current; it is formed on the basis of the interests of the self-preservative instinct" (p. 180). Even when Freud (e.g., 1940a) had given up the idea of a self-preservative instinct, he still could emphasize how it is the satisfaction of nourishment needs which produces love, and how it is to such nourishment that libidinal gratification also becomes attached. Freud (1940a) stated:

> A child's first erotic object is the mother's breast that nourishes it; love has its origin in attachment to the *satisfied* need for nourishment. (p. 188, italics mine)

But it is clear that to view love in this way, simply as reinforced attachment behavior, runs counter to evidence for the occurrence of human attachment behavior independent of such a reinforcement of nourishment (Bowlby, 1969) and actually downplays the direct importance of sexuality for love which Freud himself emphasized in other of his writings. Further, I do not think that Winnicott's solution to this problem will wash, and this is simply to redefine what Freud (1940a) meant by the mother's breast as "the first erotic object" (p. 188). Winnicott (1953) puts the matter this way:

> When it is said that the first object is the breast, the word "breast" is used, I believe, to stand for the technique of mothering as well as for the actual flesh. (p. 11)

But the quality of some immediate libidinal gratification experience with the "breast" or "flesh" is not the same thing as qualities which originate in the relationship which pertains to a "technique of mothering." It is the recognition of just this difference which enables us to conceptualize the importance of relationship matters as "mutual cueing" (Mahler, Pine, and Bergman, 1975, p. 49), whether or not the mother is "quietly available" (Mahler, Pine, and Bergman, 1975, p. 79), "consistent attitude" (Spitz, 1962, p. 99) and so forth. However, a recognition in our theory of such a difference hardly does away with the relevance of instinctual drive experience for the emergence of love. It is just this—the "technique of mothering" related to the occurrence and consequence of loving and hateful desires—which will determine whether the child will come to represent himself or herself as loving and lovable.

Nor can this complex, *inherently* dangerous situation which is love be understood by a concept of attachment behavior (Bowlby, 1969). Attachment behavior, at whatever level of animal development we study, must be tempered by a realization about how subtle the interplay can be between organism and environment with respect to any so-called fixed action pattern (Moltz, 1965). But there is no difficulty for a psychoanalytic concept of love in the fact that the young of a variety of species (e.g., Bowlby, 1969; Harlow, 1958), including Homo sapiens, is preadapted to respond with attachment behavior to a mother figure, given the occurrence of a species expectable environment (Hartmann, 1939). To use this phenomenon of attachment behavior as an argument against the importance of drive excitements for love (Bowlby, 1969) is simply to bark up the wrong tree. The dangers for which attachment behavior is preadapted are *situational and external* threats (predatory animals, absence of food, etc.) which would produce a dangerous, forced separation between child and mother. The dangers of human love are *intrinsic* to the love experience itself. Love's dangers are produced by *internal dynamics* inherent in that love relationship.

These dangers inherent in love are not only about the effects of the young child's sexual excitements upon the mother. Freud (1930a) once indicated how an individual in an intense love experience may experience anxiety because "the boundary between ego [for which we must read an individuated representation of the self] and object threatens to melt away" (p. 66). But I do maintain that this matter of individuation, as one aspect of development, is not a psychoanalytically understood drive, and that anxieties always and only are provoked by that panoply of libidinal and aggressive drives with which we are familiar, or by what I have called love and hate desires which emerge out of such drives. The young child normally will experience anxiety that his or her oral drives will deplete and/or destroy the now known to be physically separate and idealized mother. In addition, especially the young child's love-instigated desire to orally replenish, or restore, the love object normally will arouse loss of control anxiety; that is, the child is now known to him or herself as a physically separate someone who is anally gratified by the auto-regulation of all of his or her activities.

Still another source of anxiety is located within the concept formulated as a "symbiotic need" (e.g., Savitt, 1969). I say "located within" because the concept of a symbiotic need combines important matters of development and motivation which I believe are better left distinguishable. One can and should talk about the earlier sorts of oral gratification which inhere in attachment behavior (Freud, 1914c) and which occur in a matrix of nonindividuation which is part of the developmental design of Homo sapiens. Oral drives obviously remain important throughout early childhood. Further, the issue of oral gratification occurring in a symbiotic stage of development can become a source of pathological fixation. Then oral drives will provoke anxiety in a later anal period of development in which the young child now prizes the psychic pleasure obtained by his or her autonomous function as a now known and felt to be separate physical entity. Oral-drive-provoked anxieties about eating and being eaten, but now occurring in the matrix of an individuated state of consciousness, naturally will come to possess disturbing meanings about de-differentiation.[4] This is evidenced in the daily practice of any analyst; and it presents a special sort of transference experience and problem in work with those individuals who possess what I have described as a meaning disturbance. These instrinsic dangers and dynamics of love are made even more complicated by those introjective and projective processes which contribute to normal individuation (e.g., Loewald, 1962).

Altogether then, this emergent, complex biosocial desire which is love is no longer reducible simply to a matter of libidinal gratification, although its creation is intrinsically related to the occurrence of such excitement. It is also clear that love cannot be reduced to any concept of attachment behavior, although such nondrive attachment also makes its contribution to the eventual normal emergence of love.

At this point it becomes important to recognize that love implicates not only a change in the nature of the libidinal drive representation, but a similar change in the aggressive drive representation as well. Loewald (1978) at least seems to suggest some such intrinsic relationship between the emergence of love and hate when he speaks about "love relations including its opposite, hate" (p. 43), but he does not elaborate upon the meaning of this suggestion. Aggressive release, which may be considered inherently episodic or episodically produced by libidinal frustration, now also changes into a relatively permanent bio-social desire toward a love object, for which the term hate should be reserved. With hate, as with love, the object also is elevated, now, so-to-speak, "negatively" elevated. Also, with hate, the object is the least variable thing about an instinct, so long as hate exists. While we certainly consider a predominance of hate over love to be pathological, the inherent achievement in the acquisition of hate should not be ignored. It becomes plainly, but grossly pathologically, evident, for example, in the dynamically unconscious, privileged, indeed loved status accorded by a paranoid schizophrenic to his or her persecutor (Freud, 1911c), as well as in the extremely disturbed self-enhancement which always is involved in such dynamics. Another sort of equally disturbed hatred toward an enhanced love object, but now destructively turned toward the self representation, is of course what characterizes melancholia (Freud, 1917e). But references to such well-known psychopathology should not obscure the relevance of the *acquisition of hate for clinically healthy development.*

The young child's experience that he or she is able to produce hate, and so effect *distance* with the mother, is, no less than love, a signficant determinant of the acquisition of a "nuclear self" and an "independent center of initiative" (Kohut, 1977, p. 177). Indeed, it is the young child's experience that he or she can produce such distance which, in part, enables the intrinsic danger of love to individuation (Mahler, e.g., 1968) to be handled. Altogether then, the young child's experienced ability to introduce loving and hating *effects* into the mothering relationship creates an actual sense of competence, that the psychological *space* between the two, to a clinically healthy extent, is subject to the child's own regulation. This matter of a sense of regulation over psychological space with the loved one is critical for individuals who possess what I have called a meaning disturbance, and the implication of this for clinical practice especially has been developed by Bouvet (1958) with his concept of "rapprocher" (p. 211). This term of Bouvet's, "rapprocher," obviously connects up with Mahler's important concept of a rapprochement subphase (e.g., Mahler, Pine, and Bergman, 1975) with respect to the development of individuation. Mahler's important observations (see especially Mahler, Pine, and Bergman, 1975) make clear how important it is, during this rapprochement subphase of the development of individuation, that mother and child negotiate the determination of the psychological space between them in a way which leaves both with a clinically healthy sense of competence and autonomy. With respect to this, as I have said, a negotiation of hate plays an important part.

All of this is not to say that this vital issue of a negotiation of a proper space between mother and child only begins with the emergence of love and hate dynamics. Infant feeding problems (e.g., Fenichel, 1945) are, of course, a classic example of the relevance of this matter at the very beginning of the life cycle. And interesting research by Brazelton, Koslowski, and Main (1974) having to do with looking behavior between mother and infant, is also relevant in this regard. Mahler and McDevitt (1968) state, "Before clear differentiation . . . has taken place . . . behavioral phenomena seem to indicate conflicting tendencies toward differentiation and, concomitantly, toward symbiotic fusion with the object" (p. 4, and also see Spock, 1963). I believe such observation should not be equated with this emergent phenomenon of love-hate dynamics which involves (1) differentiated self and object representation, to which (2) grandiose and idealizing versus humiliating and degrading qualities now adhere, with (3) a *consciousness* (representation however immature) of various anxiety contents about the gratification experience itself, none of which is possessed by the infant. I suggest that a term used by Mahler and McDevitt (1968), "ambitendency" (p. 11), could be generalized to depict all such differentiation as contrasted to fusion tendencies prior to the emergence of love-hate dynamics.

With all of this, I also have signaled my agreement with the proposition already put forth by Bergmann (1980), namely, that love is an emergent which occurs in the "rapprochement" (Mahler, e.g., 1975, pp. 291–292) subphase of individuation. This is at least congruent with an observation made earlier by A. Freud and Burlingham (1942) that it is not until the second year of life that "the personal attachment of the child to its mother . . . comes to its *full* development" (p. 50, italics mine). I believe one can, and should say with Bergmann (1980) that love "has its origin in . . . longing . . . however dim, of the feeling state of the symbiotic phase" (p. 70 and see also Bergmann, 1971). But love immediately is contingent, as both Bergmann (1980) and Bak (1973) have stressed, upon the development of individuation. I only add a stress that love desire is an emergent which develops out of past libidinal gratification and attachment behavior occurring in a symbiotic stage of development, and these are altogether different sorts of experiences. Stated phenomenologically, romantic love desire possesses a quality we can designate as *yearning*. This sense of yearning informs us that love as a desire for a merging-closeness is active, but it is a desire which nevertheless cannot do away with representational-boundary structures (Kernberg, 1977), and this registers as a sense that our loving desire for merging-closeness will never be completely realizable. It is this, I believe, which gives clinically healthy, romantic love its bittersweet quality.

But there is another important perspective to be added with respect to the development of the meaning apparatus. This is that love requires the achievement by the young child of a functional grade in experience between what I have called actuality and not-real (playful) grandiosity and idealization. Love is a prime example of how, as Freud (1914c) once put it, "where libido is concerned man [is] incapable of giving up a satisfaction he had once enjoyed" (p. 94). Freud, in this same material, talks about how man can create a "substitute" (p. 94) for this lost gratification of the symbiotic period. But I believe a term like "substitute" may obscure the developmental achievement which is love (and hate); that is, it at least leans toward the fallacy (Hartmann and Lowenstein, 1962) of equating an emergent psychic structure, which produces new psychic function and content, with a genetic determinant of such a developmental emergent.[5]

I believe that my contention that the bio-social desires of both love and hate represent an emergent development from instinctual drives is congruent with a statement by Freud I will cite in a moment. The context for these comments by Freud clearly is about love and hate desires throughout the life cycle. But Freud here uses the term "total ego." I will be consistent with my own earlier comments if I reread "total ego" to mean a whole personality organization. Then, these desires of love and hate cannot be comprehended as ego activities in earlychildhood, but as processes attributable to psychic structures which are not yet integrated into a whole personality organization. Freud's (1915c) statement is this:

> We might at a pinch say of an instinct that it "loves" the object toward which it strives for purposes of satisfaction; but to say that an instinct "hates" an object strikes us as odd. Thus we become aware that the attitudes of love and hate cannot be made use of for the relations of instincts to their objects, but are reserved for the relations of the *total ego* to objects. (Freud, 1915c, p. 137)

But I do not want these comments about the emergent nature of love and hate to lead to any mistaken conclusion that I believe this "does away" with the importance of psycho-sexual libidinal and aggressive drives. Psycho-sexual, libidinal, and aggressive drives are never "done away." They always remain the vital sources of human experience and behavior for Freudian psychoanalytic theory. What I want to stress is that when I speak about the emergent nature of love and hate, I simply mean by this new characteristics which now inhere in the representation of various libidinal and aggressive drive experiences, and which have an important consequence for human behavior and experience. But love and hate, taken as quite general concepts, never do justice to clinically normal or abnormal individual vicissitudes. There are, dynamically, many kinds of love, and different sorts of hate, directed toward either self or object representation, and we only can understand this variety via an examination of dynamically unconscious, instinctual drives which support these bio-social desires. This kind of examination, of course, is exactly what constitutes a significant aspect of psychoanalysis as a clinical practice.[6]

We consider, psychoanalytically, that some degree of hatred will exist together with romance and tender longing toward the love object, and this we express in our concept of ambivalence, something which Freud (1915b) once soberly called a "law" (p. 293) of life. But if I am correct that love and hate in themselves are emergent developmental achievements, then ambivalence also should be reserved as a special term for such achievements. In this way I can understand Winnicott's (1954a) statement that ambivalence is to be understood "as an achievement in emotional development" (p. 263). But also, in keeping with the developmental perspective about splitting and denial adopted in this investigation, it is important theoretically to distinguish a defensive splitting-ambivalence in the young child or adult (such as is grossly, pathologically evident in paranoia or melancholia) from a clinically normal and healthy ambivalence, which implicates a potential for the achievement of integration of love and hate desires in self and object representation structures.

A further, important question now immediately arises. How does the clinically healthy young child accomplish an integration of such ambivalence? And, by definition, the idea of such an integration carries a congruent idea about the acquisition of self and object constancy (Hartmann, 1952). It is a commonplace observation that a clinically healthy child will show a steady, progressive, and natural reduction in ambivalence from the intense negativism of the eighteen month to two-year-old.[7] But the meaning apparatus of the young child throughout this entire period does not enable the acquistion of self or object representation which can actually possess an integration of such impelling, contradictory, and conflictual qualities of love and hate. In fact, exactly because the young child's meaning apparatus cannot structure a self or object representation which possesses an integration of such diverse love-hate qualities, this same apparatus in part is responsible for the awesomeness with which the young child will experience ambivalence: Hate does momentarily "destroy" what is "good" (and vice versa) with respect to either self or object representation, inasmuch as no meaning structure exists than can integrate such diverse, compelling qualities.[8] Further, the meaning apparatus of the young child is not yet one in which object idealizing and self-aggrandizing representations are differentiated structurally from self or object referent actuality (Piaget, e.g., 1945). Therefore, cycles of idealization and grandiosity versus disillusionment and humiliation with self or other take on a particular and unique urgency even for a clinically healthy young child. And yet, a progressive increase in tolerance for such ambivalence creating discrepancy is a regular sign of development in the clinically healthy young child, and we must attempt to account for it.

Now one can, if one wishes, take a theoretical position that there is evident already in early childhood an achievement of a "whole person" (Winnicott, 1954a, p. 264) or "unit status" (Winnicott, 1954a, p. 266) or "whole object relations" (Winnicott, 1954a, p. 272) or "object constancy" (Mahler, Pine, and Bergman, 1975, p. 162) or a "coherent self" (Kohut, 1977, p. 93), or a "cohesive self" (Tolpin, 1972, p. 316) or "integration of a whole" (Stolorow and Lachmann, 1980, p. 122). But it must be kept in mind that the representation-making capabilities of the young child do not enable the achievement of either self or object representations which actually are a structural integration of impellingly different love-hate qualities. What then can such terminology mean? It can mean something in terms of another felicitous term produced by Winnicott (1954a)—"holding" (p. 269). Loving acts enable the young child to acquire self representation quality as someone who can "hold"—in the sense of hold *on to* or *bring back* or *make*—the "good" mother (representation) once again "full" after a loving or hateful attack (and thus secure himself or herself for a future fulfillment). But this can only occur if the mother, by her vividly acknowledged pleasure and response to the child's love acts, enables the child to acquire representation as someone who can, *in actuality*, reproduce the "good" and "full" object (representation) lost because of loving (assault) gratification and/or hate (Winnicott, 1954a).[9]

Jacobson (1957) asks us to imagine the following commonplace example:

> If little Johnny after a temper tantrum assures his mother that now bad Johnny is gone and good Johnny is here again, he is fully aware that it is he who was angry and who now feels loving again. But he still experiences and expresses the change of his thoughts and feelings, of his own state and behavior, in concretistic, personifying and generalizing terms of a disappearance of bad and a reappearance of good Johnny. (p. 125)

Indeed, "little Johnny," or an adult (e.g., Kernberg, 1966) who employs splitting and denial can remember the angry experience. But no psychic structure exists by which one can represent the self to be objectively both the hateful and the loving person. Therefore "little Johnny" (I would say lovingly) can reassure his mother that "good Johnny" has returned only if a "good enough" (Winnicott, e.g., 1953, p. 237) mother "holds the situation" (Winnicott, 1954a, p. 267). This mother who "holds" is the mother who maintains through such hatred an adequate feeling of love and devotion. Such a mother who "holds" waits for, recognizes, pleasurably accepts, and *does not call into question* her child's love gift gesture on account of previous expressions of loving assault and/or hatred (Winnicott, 1954a).[10] I believe that what is equally important, in light of my earlier comments about the developmental achievement of hate, is what this "good enough" (Winnicott, 1953, p. 237) mother does in response to the child's intention to reproduce a hateful (bad) self or object representation. The "good enough" mother here is one who, while remaining potentially available for future love, nevertheless demonstrates by her response that she has been affected, so that distance for the moment has been created between her child and herself.[11] Altogether then, this mother who "holds" enables the young child increasingly to acquire a self representation as someone who can hold onto, i.e., determine either a "good" or "bad" self and object representation, and so control the psychological space between mother and child to a clinically healthy extent. It is exactly this which increases the young child's tolerance for ambivalence and accounts for its gradual, observable diminishment in normal child development.

These comments about ambivalence naturally have an implication for our psychoanalytic concept of object and self constancy (Hartmann, 1952). Mahler (1968), in an earlier formulation about the psychoanalytic concept of object constancy, stated the following:

> Solid integration, in which there is a blending and synthesis of "good" and "bad" mother images, even in normal development, is not achieved . . . during the separation-individuation phase. . . . *With the advent of the latency period* the child should clearly perceive and recognize not only that the mother is separate and complex, but that other important love objects and he himself are separate and complex as well. (pp 46–47, italics mine)

But in a later communication, Mahler, Pine, and Bergman (1975) state the following:

> But the constancy of the object implies more than the maintenance of the representation of the absent love object. It also implies the unifying of the"good" and "bad" object into one whole representation.
>
> The slow establishment of emotional object constancy is a complex and multidetermined process involving all aspects of psychic development.
>
> It is only after object constancy is well on its way, which according to our conceptualization does not occur before the third year, that the mother during her physical absence can be substituted for, at least in part, by the presence of a reliable internal image that remains relatively stable" (p. 110).

The theoretical problem is, as Mahler, Pine, and Bergman (1975) describe it, that the concept of object constancy first appears to implicate the acquisition of self versus object representation, but also it is used to refer to a further development in integration, the "unifying of the 'good' and 'bad' object into one whole representation."

But I believe that what creates this theoretical problem is another theoretical issue which stands in the background, and here I repeat some of my initial comments that psychoanalysis as a developmental psychology must be able theoretically to document both change and continuity in the life cycle. If, as has been suggested (Kaplan, 1972, 1978; Mahler, Pine, and Bergman, 1975), one speaks about a degree of object constancy, then the object constancy concept is being used to document continuity in the life cycle. But we are still left with the theoretical documentation of emergent change which, just as much as continuity, characterizes human development. I believe that the concept of object constancy should be reserved for the documentation of such an emergent change, which I think is more in keeping with Hartmann's (1952) introduction of this concept. Another felicitous term introduced by Mahler (e.g., 1968), individuation, then can be used to talk about the history of the articulation of boundaries for psychic structures throughout the life cycle. This will eliminate what otherwise can appear as an inconsistency in Mahler's important observations. A psychoanalytic concept of object constancy then will not be burdened to mean two quite different achievements that are made at different points in the life cycle: The acquisition of self versus object representation constitutes a first achievement; the young child now knows and feels that he or she and the mother have two separate bodies which exist both within and without contexts of drive activation. The acquistion of a "complex" self and object representation, which is an authentic, conceptual integrate of "good" and "bad," is another emergence in individuation for which we can reserve the terms object and self constancy. So understood, object constancy is not something a child can acquire until mid-latency, and it implicates a further achievement in *boundary articulation with respect to an internalization of self-esteem regulation* (see Steingart, 1969). A further, theoretical documentation remains to be written about the life cycle history of this articulation of boundaries for psychic structures, i.e., individuation.[12]

Ambivalence, and a steady growth in its toleration, is, of course, critical for the eventual achievement of object constancy (Hartmann, 1952). However, clinically, a normally developing young child's tolerance for ambivalence is to be understood simply and wholly to be a function of a growing competence and confidence to "hold on to" or "make"—i.e., determine—the occurrences of love and hate representations of variated ambivalent experience. Later, with further emotional development and maturity in the meaning apparatus achieved in latency, love versus hate ambivalence now can become authentically structured into a single whole self and object representation. It is this achievement which I take to be characteristic of neurotic psychopathology, that is, individuals who do not possess what I have described as a meaning disturbance as pathological play.

But we also have in our literature a concept of a "post-ambivalent" (Abraham, 1924) object relationship. I want now to examine how certain further potentialities for meaning production relate to this idea of post-ambivalence and, as well, to social ideology.

7

Further Development of Real and Not-Real Meaning in the Individual and Social Ideology—Paradoxical Creation

I will begin with some description of Abraham's (1924) concept of "post-ambivalent" (p. 496). I indicate how a comprehension of certain further development in procedures for meaning production can illuminate this concept, and I term such further development the emergence of paradoxical creation. I then can show how this concept of paradoxical creation can help us to understand certain eternal subject matter in any group (social) ideology, and this is related to the arts and sciences, religion, and philosophy, as well as to mythology. With regard to mythology, I take up especially the mythology of love experience.

If the concept of a "post-ambivalent" object relationship has a psychological significance, and I think it does, then we must refer such a concept to a still later point in the life cycle. I believe such a capability for a post-ambivalence is part and parcel of what Blos (e.g., 1967) calls the "second individuation" (p. 162) of adolescence, and, in part, this is enabled by the emergence of another type of "thought structure" (Freud, 1900a, p. 542).[1] In part because of further growth in the meaning apparatus, together, of course, with psychodynamic, object relationship, etc., maturity, the meaning of a human relationship can now be fully known and felt to be humanly devised. Then, any particular kind of love, hate, or ambivalence is no longer experienced as something necessarily given in a human relationship, the way we know and feel this to be the case when we are young, or even older, children. Another aspect of this is to say that what can occur as part of the resolution of this "second individuation" in adolescence is a new kind of integration of experience indexed as real in relationship to experience which is known and felt to be imaginatively not-real. In order to develop these thoughts further, I must briefly recapitulate, and then enlarge upon, some previous material.

I have described how the acquisition of a capability for a representation of ambivalence, which is authentically structured as such, is in part determined by an emergence of mature meaning structures characteristic of mid-latency, and in particular with respect to self and object representation (Steingart, 1969). I also already have described how a meaning apparatus which can so organize diverse, impelling, prototype-image love and hate qualities into an authentically integrated representation (concept) also must possess full differentiation of any symbol from a reality signified by such a symbol. This has an important consequence for idealization of the object as well as grandiose enhancement of the self. Idealized and grandiose content now is known and felt to be not-real aspects of experience which can enrich clinically healthy life with "imaginative living" (Winnicott, 1953, p. 14). This is in contrast to not-real experience which is "alienating" (Freud, 1911b, p. 218) from reality due to neurotic conflict, or what I have called a meaning disturbance that "perverts" reality consideration altogether. I believe that to look at the development of idealization in this way, from the viewpoint of growth in the meaning apparatus, clarifies Freud's (1912d) statement that a man "must have surmounted his respect" (p. 186) for a woman in order to be able to love in a clinically healthy, free way. In the same way, this viewpoint clarifies what Balint (1948) means by a concept of mature "genital love [which] requires a constant testing of reality," (p. 37) as well as Kernberg's (1974d) statement that there exists "an idealization more sophisticated than that characteristic of primitive splitting operations" (p. 749; also see 1974c). Elsewhere (Steingart, 1969), I have described love as having to do with "standards of drive gratification" (p. 292). Such idealization matures in part because of growth in the meaning apparatus, and such a meaning apparatus determines and is determined by overall differentiating and integrating processes which produce a mature (id, ego, superego) personality organization. Concepts similar to what I have just described for love can be generalized (Steingart, 1969) to include ideals of the psychic system ego (e.g., competence, management, etc.), as well as the superego (e.g., honesty, virtue, etc.). The point here is that, in clinically normal and neurotic personality development, all such gratifying ideal or grandiose content is now known and experienced to be special, at least potentially enriching, symbols which, nevertheless, are firmly differentiated from reality.

I will consider that ideals of "imaginative living" (Winnicott, 1953, p. 14) use what Piaget (e.g., 1947) calls a "concrete operation" (p. 137) type of conceptual structure. I have indicated that this means that the existence of these ideas is now fully differentiated from an experience indexed as real and for which such ideals can provide a special grandiose and idealized enrichment. Linguistic or other symbolic vehicles which express such ideals are not believed to magically control events. And inasmuch as such imaginative content is structured as an authentic concept, idealization and grandiose representation now can possess a mature order of stability unknown to the young child. But the existence of such imaginative, grandiose, and idealized representation, even though it is so differentiated and integrated with respect to reality, requires the constant supporting occurrence of the same real event or relationship for its maintenance as a vital source of enrichment for the older child or adult.[2]

The further development in imaginative, not-real content which can take place occurs, in part, because of what Piaget (e.g., 1947) calls "formal operations" (pp. 147–150) representation. All representation—including therefore gratifying ideal and grandiose imaginative content—now is known to be humanly made. Piaget (1964) once described this as follows:

> Thought [is] raised to be the second power. Concrete thinking is the representation of a possible action, and formal thinking is the representation of a representation of possible action.
>
> Formal opeartions provide thinking with an entirely new ability that detaches and liberates thinking from concrete reality and permits it to build its own reflections and theories. (p. 63)

This should not be taken to mean that the referential relationship between such imaginative representations and reality need be experienced as tenuous or confused, which we would take to be the case with psychopathology. But this does mean that such imaginative content which is now known and felt to be humanly devised—created—is not necessarily made secure by any actual, real event as is the case with ideals of "imaginative living" (Winnicott, 1953, p. 14). An obvious illustration of this is the emergence of a representation of the idea of infinity which inherently is not secured in any event indexed as real.

But my interest is in what such a development of a meaning apparatus implies for personal life experience and behavior. One implication is something to which I already have alluded with the concept of post-ambivalence. It is important to clarify what I am doing with this concept of post-ambivalence in terms of the meaning apparatus perspective used in this investigation. It is not at all that love, hate, ambivalence in any way become transcended as human experience. Once achieved in development, love, hate, and ambivalence never can be made to go away. But any particular meaning of love, hate, and ambivalence now is known and felt to be humanly devised and not necessarily secured by any particular reality about a relationship. One immediately is reminded about how adolescence, at least in the modern, industrial society, can be characterized by a natural turmoil of this sort about the meaning of human life; in fact, this further development in procedures for meaning production, which is a necessary but insufficient condition for the emergence of such post-ambivalence, does arise in adolescence (e.g., Piaget, 1964.)[3]

The imaginative construction enabled by this new development in meaning production amounts to a new relationship between real and not-real experience and is inherently in the nature of a paradox. For this reason, I call this new kind of imaginative representation paradoxical creation.[4] Any idea, whether indexed to be real or not-real, is now felt and known to be humanly created—an invention—and as such there is no necessary basis for such content in experience. Imaginative construction now can move into the foreground of life experience in a way that provides it with a special sort of status, and we first become capable of this at adolescence (Steingart, 1969). Imaginative construction now can enjoy a preeminence with respect to reality, and, paradoxically, this makes it poignant, critical, and urgent that one discover a referent for such imaginative construction with experience indexed as real. If this is not achieved, we have either madness (e.g., Kris, 1952) or what I have termed a meaning disturbance. What apparently can happen is that such an advance in imaginative construction enables an individual to now represent and find reference with respect to the basic functions of the psychic systems in themselves. But we conceptualize these basic functions of the psychic systems to constitute the essentials of any individual personality organization. Therefore, imaginative construction about such subject matter will be statements about what is the eternal human condition. Looked at from the viewpoint of a particular society or group to which an individual belongs, such statements constitute various forms of expression of that society's ideology.

The basic function of the psychic system superego is the setting up of ideals as well as the registration of discrepancy between experience indexed as real self representation and ideal self representation (Hartmann, Kris, and Lowenstein, 1947). It is, of course, the purpose of religion to supply us with such ideals. At the same time, it is interesting to realize that what characterizes contemporary religion is an understanding of how such ideals are paradoxical creations, and this expresses itself in the existential crisis literature which is such a prominent feature of modern religious writing. Thus, we have Etienne Gilson, who reinterprets Thomasism in terms of a "notion of being" (1957, p. 629). Tillich (1952) speaks about how the act of accepting meaninglessness is "itself an act of faith" (p. 680). Martin Buber (1947) states that a secure belief about the universe as a home created by God for humans is no longer comprehensible. This is so, says Buber (1947), because now an idea of infinite "must be included in the image of the universe—which is a paradox, for an image . . . is limited, yet the unlimited itself must enter the image." (p. 700) Freud (1927c), of course, was alive to such contemporary stirrings in religious thought. However, Freud (1927c) chose to argue a case against religious belief with an idea of religious belief modeled after what I have described as play (or illusion). That is, Freud considered that the only authentic definition of religion must involve a belief in the personage of God, Heaven, redemption, and so forth. Freud therefore looked forward to the day when human kind could dispense with such religious belief altogether. But if religion is the institutionalized expression of superego (ego-ideal) structure and function, Freud's belief that religion is not necessary at least implies that we can theoretically imagine a mature personality organization which does not possess a psychic system superego. But I think such a view is mistaken, and I here agree with Stein (1966), who states that we cannot regard the psychic system superego as some sort of "vestigial structure" (p. 294). Loewald (1978), in particular, has expressed the realization that it is ego-ideal content and function of the psychic system superego which is "the representative of futurity. It represents the care and concern we have for ourselves, in past and present, as continuing on into a future that is to be shaped" (p. 23; see also Loewald, 1962b). Stated in other words, the psychic system superego is a structure which possesses function and content according to a future mode. Only if such a future mode is operative within a personality can there be value, ambition, purpose, etc., which support the workings of healthy narcissism (Kohut, e.g., 1971, 1977). These ideas of contemporary religious literature, therefore, can be understood as paradoxical creation, that is, not-real constructions which nevertheless illuminate a necessary function and content for mature personality organization. Certainly, one can grant that the idea of Heaven, and so forth, is some kind of literal concretization of a perpetual future mode. But another view would emphasize a "relative" autonomy of the psychic system superego (Hartmann and Lowenstein, 1962), how imaginative religious ideals as paradoxical creations contribute to this achievement, and how contemporary religious literature can be regarded as an expression of this development.

The essential function of the psychic system ego is relations with reality (Hartmann, Kris, and Lowenstein, 1947), and it is the business of art, science, and philosophy to comprehend and construct this reality for us. But it is characteristic of art, science, and philosophy to place in the foreground, each in their own way, imaginative paradoxical creations which thus take distance from and yet illuminate reality for us.

Art, genuine art, is neither childish play, nor magic, and certainly it is not the making of illusion, which denies reality considerations for some pathological purpose with regard to self and object esteem regulation and/or emotional survival in a core area of representation. In whatever medium art may be expressed, it is intended to illuminate what is real. Great art produces, as Keats put it, "a fellowship with essence." Kris (1952) indicates that art is a "type of [I would say, psychic system ego] problem solving behavior" (p. 251). Dewey (1935) expresses this idea in the following manner.

> Through art, meanings of objects that are otherwise dumb, inchoate, restricted, and resisted are clarified and concentrated, and not by thought working laboriously upon them, nor by escape into a world of mere sense, but by the creation of a new experience. (p. 992)

Notice Dewey's illusion to "meanings. . .that are. . .resisted" as well as his contention that art is not "mere sense." In this way, a philosopher indicates his belief that authentic art represents imagination which now paradoxically acts in the service of the revelation of reality. I believe that Freud (1911b) had a similar idea in mind when he described how the artist can "mold his fantasies into thoughts of a new kind which are valued by men as reflections of reality" (p. 224).

However, while Freud (1911b) could thus describe art as a "reconciliation between the two [reality and pleasure] principles" (p. 224), he never would formulate science in such a manner. Science, for Freud (1911b) "comes nearest to succeeding in that conquest [of the pleasure principle]" (p. 223), and artistic, paradoxical creation never acquires such a status in Freud's writing. But is this true of science and its attendant logical reasoning? Piaget (1947) himself calls logic a kind of "morality of thinking" (p. 163), which already suggests an imaginative idealization of such thought processes. Actually, strictly logical reasoning does not even accurately completely characterize the thinking of scientists at work (e.g., Kaplan, 1964). But more to the point is the relevance of imaginative, paradoxical creation for scientific theory construction. Science, Whitehead (1925) reminds us, is founded upon "a faith in the order of nature" . . . (p. 20). Contemporary scientific theory contains hypothetical constructions which qualify as paradoxical creations, impossible in principle to ever be substantiated by real appearances, but yet responsive to and able to illuminate what James (1890) once called "irreducible and stubborn facts" (p. 225). The fact that scientific, imaginative, theoretical constructions, unlike art, philosophy, and religion, are evaluated by certain public, verifiable procedures ought not to obscure this issue. The point here is that any hypothetical construction of science involves such paradoxical creation, and this is exactly the call to arms raised by that modern philosophy known as logical positivism (e.g., Schlick, 1938). The fact that such a philosophical movement as logical positivism arose is itself evidence for my contention that it is in the nature of scientific theory to be paradoxical creation.[5]

Finally, I want to examine imagination as paradoxical creation with respect to the psychic system id, which has to do with the "basic needs of man and his striving for gratification" (Hartmann, Kris, and Lowenstein, 1947, p. 15). But in order to do this I must again return to Freud's (1920g) *Beyond the Pleasure Principle* monograph. I am once again in touch with Freud's (1920g) ideas of a life and death instinct. Why, to return once again to Freud's (1920g) words, apply the "predicate instinctual" (p. 36) to these ideas of a life and death instinct? And what has this to do with my intention to investigate imaginative, paradoxical creation with respect to our construct of a psychic system id? Just this, that the bedrock, the *sine qua non*, of Freudian psychoanalytic theory is the body's involvement in human existence. No contribution of Freud's is greater than his conceptualization for us about how our bodies become involved in human behavior and experience through the vicissitudes and development of libidinal and aggressive drives. But instinctual, libidinal, and aggressive drives, in addition to what I have called love and hate bio-social desires which are emergent developments from such drives, altogether constitute the essentials of motivational theory for Freudian psychoanalysis. Libidinal and aggressive drives, as well as love and hate desires, remain theoretical psychological constructs which thus properly belong to a psychoanalytic psychology of human behavior and experience. But then, once again, why apply the "predicate instinctual" (Freud, 1920g,

p. 36) to these matters of life and death which humans share with other life forms? I believe Freud (1920g) applied "the predicate instinctual" (p. 36) because the man who created dynamic psychology, and who in particular created a psychology which comprehends the body's motivational involvement in human experience and behavior, now wanted to recognize what can be called the body's "ultimate" contribution. What else is this "ultimate" contribution of our body but life and death?

How and why it is that humans, together with other life forms, first evolve and develop and then decay and die, is not, I think, a subject matter proper for a psychoanalytic psychology. But it is only about one organism—human—that we can ask, nevertheless, a certain question about the effects of an *awareness* of life and death, which thus is properly psychological. This is, whether a human being indeed really lives—and this means develops—ever more complex, tension-maintaining and using psychic structure, function, and content even with the realization of death (Erikson, 1950; Kohut, 1971; Levinson et al., 1958). But I believe this enters into awareness as a psychological phenomenon only at adolescence and this, in part, is due to the still further advance of the meaning apparatus into what Piaget (e.g., 1927) calls "formal operations" (p. 147) representation (see also Steingart, 1969). It should be clear from my earlier comments about the emergence of a meaning apparatus, that such a knowledge about a life that must end in death is not possible for a young child. Certainly a young child may suffer the loss, say, of a loved parent or friend. It is true enough that even a young child, in such a circumstance, can experience loss and will react with depression (e.g., Furman, 1964). But meaning for a young child is egocentric—including the meaning of death—and any death will be related by a young child to some egocentric interpretation concerning his or her own life. And even an older, latency child cannot know and feel about *impersonal* death, i.e., that death is the same for us all, however one concretely has lived one's life.

I believe that Freud himself suspected that his concepts of a life and death instinct actually might be paradoxical, imaginative constructions rather than motivational concepts for psychoanalysis as a scientific psychology. Freud (1920g) said the following:

> If we are to die ourselves, and first to lose in death those who are dearest to us, it is easier to submit to a remorseless law of nature, to the sublime *Avάγxn* [Necessity], than to a chance which might perhaps have been escaped. It may be, however, that this belief in the eternal necessity of dying is only another of those illusions which we have created *'um die Schwere des Daseins zu ertragen'* [to bear the burden of existence]. (p. 45)[6]

But if I believe that Freud, at this moment, is saying to us that these ideas of the life and death instinct are paradoxical creations, they are not examples of paradoxical creations as scientific, theoretical constructs, and these life and death instinct concepts are neither artistic, nor religious, nor philosophical constructions. But then, to what category of paradoxical imaginative construction do they belong? I suggest that these ideas of the life and death instinct belong to another category of imaginative construction we call myth. Indeed, in the passage just cited, Freud refers to the Greek god of necessity. I now will regard these ideas of the life and death instincts as myth-making—one can easily imagine dramatic and fabulously powerful life and death figures contesting on a stage which is the entire scope of human behavior and experience. But I believe that such myth also is paradoxical creation. What is more real—eternal—about human existence than that first life and then death come, however we live?

I now can propose a generalization: All myth, including myth in a contemporary society saturated with scientific outlook, is in the nature of paradoxical creation. Myth records, in idealizing and grandiose terms, instinctual characteristics of human experience and behavior which in fact are eternal. Kluckhohn (1959) states this as follows:

> Their persistence [myths] cannot be understood except on the hypothesis that these images have a special congeniality for the human mind. It suggests that the interaction of a certain kind of biological apparatus in a certain kind of physical world with some inevitabilities of the human condition (the helplessness of infants, two parents of different sex, etc.) bring about some regularities in the formation of imaginative productions, of powerful images. (p. 49)

And Campbell (1959) describes this in the following manner:

> Shall we find, in tracing our mythological themes to their points of origin, that these can be identified in discoverable strata of the well of history? Or shall we find, rather, when the bottom of the well has been reached and even broached, that the origin or ground of myth will not have been attained? If the latter, then we shall be justified in asserting that at least some of the archetypes on which the wonder tales and religions of mankind have been founded derive not from any fund of human experience in time but from some structuring principle antecedent to history—or even the cause of history; namely, the form of the psyche itself, as a function of the biology of the human body. (p. 22)

I now must relate my comments about myth to a valuable distinction introduced into our literature by Loewald (1978). This has to do with how an individual can experience a sense of eternality—which is without any time index, outside, so-to-speak, time altogether—versus a sense of everlastingness, a limitless future, which remains essentially within a time framework. What I am saying is that myth articulates, in grandiose and idealizing terms, what is eternal about human experience and behavior. Freud (1915b) stated that, for each of us, our dynamic unconscious behaves "as if it were immortal" (p. 296). But frequently he also expressed the view that the dynamic unconscious was without any time index (e.g., Freud, 1915e). I believe that the term "immortal" in the just cited quotation should be understood to mean eternal, i.e., without time. Myth documents what is so eternal about human experience and behavior. The destructive as well as grandiose and idealizing terms of myth not only elevate some characteristic of human existence, but also, in some manner, this elevation accomplishes a "suspension" of such a characteristic into a realm of experience without time. It was the ancient Greeks who took the revolutionary step of enlarging human consciousness by a complete portrayal of their gods and goddesses as humans (e.g., Hamilton, 1930, 1942). But the Greeks did not accomplish by this only a glorification of the human experience and behavior. The Greeks, by this elevation of their mortal human lives into the lives of gods and goddesses, made a statement about what is the actual eternality of certain essential features of human experience and behavior. I do not claim that only mythic material can be used to have such a sense of eternality about human experience and behavior. Clearly it is possible to have such a sense of contemplative eternality about matters of ideals, values, and purpose which we theoretically understand to be the essential function of the psychic system superego. In the same way, with a sense of contemplative eternality, we can experience the natural laws of science, the rules of logic, works of art, as well as philosophical ideas, all of which we recruit conceptually to the basic function of the psychic system ego to establish relations with reality. But myth gloriously records in a more direct way the hurly-burly, libidinal and aggressive, *instinctual* aspect of the spectacle of the human scene, and is in this way especially responsive to our dynamically unconscious belief that we are eternal.[7]

Myth, as Arlow (1961) puts it, "is a special form of shared fantasy" (p. 375). I suggest that it is myth's paradoxical creation that makes it so special. But this special "shared fantasy" (Arlow, 1961, p. 375) which is myth, in a modern scientific society obviously cannot possess the same sort of power which derives from a cohesive ideology present in antiquity, or some present-day, pre-literate society. Concern over the absence of such cohesive ideology is thus understandable. Eliot (1922), for example, in his powerful voice, claims contemporary modern society to be a "wasteland" (p. 37) with a "heap of broken images" (p. 38). And Yeats (1924) contends that individuals who exist in such a contemporary, modern society can no longer believe, and hence feel like the "more sensitive people of ancient times" (p. 51). Murray's (1960) seriously intentioned as well as eloquent call for a new, powerful mythology which somehow will make use of contemporary life is thus understandable. However this may be, it is clear that in a modern society who shall share in what mythic experience is largely an individual affair based upon individual interests and capabilities. Modern myth-making is something which spontaneously develops about a life event of some actual individual; the event and the individual then accrue imaginative, paradoxically creative content. For example, Babe Ruth audaciously points to the center field wall and thus signals where he intends to hit a home run. Amelia Earhart dares to fly the Pacific Ocean in a single-engine plane. Joe Louis, in his return bout with Max

Schmeling, knocks out Schmeling in two minutes, four seconds, in the first round. Astronauts dare to fly and land upon the moon. Myth-making, then, both elevates and transforms such individual happenings into eternal features of human experience which exist "outside" of time because such experience must and will forever be pertinent to every human being's instinctual life: the confrontation and conquest of feared danger, the exultant overcoming of ignominious defeat, the determination to challenge one's fate in the face of an indifferent universe, and so forth.

Myth-making also accomplishes a certain coalescence of individual and event, an individual-event is created which becomes *legendary* and is passed on from one generation to the next. Sometimes, this legend can comprise an individual's entire life cycle. It is some kind of irony that Freud, who himself shunned such legendary idealization (Kohut, 1977), is himself such a subject for myth-making. Freud (1927c) was a man who said, "The voice of the intellect is a soft one, but it does not rest till it has gained a hearing" (p. 53). It is hardly news to observe that Freud identified himself with the human desire to know (in scientific procedure and logical reasoning), as well as the responsibility to acknowledge and face the reality about human beings revealed by such a stance (e.g., 1915e, 1927c, 1930a). But notice that in this citation Freud shows his faith in the eventual victory of intellect (which is true, of course, for any committed scientist), as well as his identification with what he believes will be the eternal working of such intellect ("It does not rest").

Finally, I want to consider a particular mythic figure from antiquity, and in so doing, I return to considerations about love. I believe this mythic contribution tells us about something which is eternal about love desire for Homo sapiens, and that what is so said is congruent with the concept of love developed earlier in this investigation.

We are accustomed each year, on February 14, Saint Valentine's Day, to see portrayals of the cherub god Eros, or as he is also called, Cupid, wielding his arrows of love desire from which none can escape. Balint (1938) already has pointed out how a favorite subject for sculpture in Greek antiquity is the triumph of Eros over the greatest god, Zeus himself, as Zeus is led behind the triumphal chariot, smiling but in chains. But why should such a powerful god as Eros, such a significant human desire as love, be portrayed as such a young child? Balint's (1938) contention that Eros is never portrayed as a mature, sexual man is incorrect. It is true that Eros is never portrayed as a mature sexual man and partner for his mother Aphrodite. But Eros is, nevertheless, portrayed as a mature heterosexual man in other contexts in Greek art, for example, in the famous love story between Eros and Psyche (see, for example, Schlam, 1976). But why is this so? Why does such different representation—cherub versus mature heterosexual man—coexist for the mythic figure of love, and as far as I can determine for no other Greek god?[8]

Balint (1938) suggests that the cherub representation of Eros is to be interpreted as pregenital sexuality, which enters into adult heterosexuality as forepleasure. Following this approach, one could speak about Cupid as child versus Eros as man, and so thus represent differences between forepleasure and genital pleasure in adult heterosexuality. While such an interpretation is plausible, it strikes me as a quite literal meaning of manifest content, as does an obvious interpretation about arrow-like, phallic, infantile, instinctual drives wielded by the god of love. However, by Balint's (1938) own account, infantile sexuality altogether, and this would include its involvement as forepleasure in adult sexuality, is a "relatively simple mechanism [and] strictly speaking, sexless" (p. 204) with regard to the representation of one's adult sexual identity. If so, then why should this sexless identity kind of infantile forepleasure, portrayed as a cherub, be able to exert such an irresistible effect and have such great power to bring about adult, heterosexual love?

I want to suggest another interpretation which derives from what love is like for us from the meaning apparatus perspective developed in this investigation. Recall that for the young child the not-real grandiose and idealized representation of the self and other, as well as the exalted status of the libidinal drive itself, all of which inhere in romantic love, are not fully differentiated from actuality. If these special characteristics of love's meaning only inhere in a young child's love, it makes sense that the powerful attraction of such a state of experience should be portrayed by a god of love represented as a young child. End-pleasure (orgasm) now can be understood as a clinically normal, physical "consummation" of meaning about such idealized, grandiose, and exalted representation. I believe what I have just said is akin to but not identical with Eissler's (1958) important idea that "one of the ego functions of orgasm is to ascertain an incontrovertible truth" (p. 239) that one exists. Nydes's (1950) comment that experience at masturbatory climax has "hallucinatory quality" (p. 306) also is close to but not identical with the view I express. I would say that the meaning of one's existence at such a climactic moment is grandiose with respect to self, idealized with respect to the object, and exalted in terms of the libidinal drive experience itself, all of this experienced as momentarily real, like intense play. Notice how we will say "Let's make love," or we will use the term "love-making," or some allied term. We do not ordinarily use such a word "make" when we anticipate a sexual encounter which will be essentially devoid of romance. What I am saying is that with erotic but also romantic love-making, a momentum develops for de-differentiation between real and not-real in the meaning apparatus. When we make love, and have good orgasm, we momentarily become as gods and goddesses. "The earth moved," (p. 174) Maria finally acknowledges to the old woman Pilar, and here she describes her love-making with the American Roberto, in Hemingway's (1921) *For Whom the Bell Tolls.* For Roberto also, "the earth moved," and he later realizes that Pilar's insistence that Maria reveal this experience "wasn't evil. It was only wanting to keep her hold on life. To keep it through Maria" (p. 176). An area of experience ultimately is located, with good mutual orgasm in erotic and romantic love-making, in which there is no longer anything which can be called a representation of self or other. All that exists is the experience itself in its overwhelming immediacy and majesty.

Such adult love-making naturally constitutes a body of sublime experience which is lost each time we return to experience structured as real versus not-real (even "imaginative living" [Winnicott, 1953, p. 14]), and against such sublime experience customary reality may suffer by comparison, dependent, of course, upon the presence or absence of psychopathology. I believe that such a meaning apparatus perspective on adult love-making experience is a useful supplement to our understanding of genital sexuality. For example, it is now an accepted observation (e.g., Lichtenstein, 1970) that certain narcissistic and borderline people who are not believed to have reached what we mean theoretically by genital sexuality, with mature object relations, nevertheless possess an ease in achieving a fulfilling orgasm with erotic love-making. A customary and certainly important dynamic explanation about such individuals who are women is that the vagina, here, in the dynamic unconscious, functions as a mouth which eats through intercourse. But from the meaning apparatus viewpoint used in this investigation, another consideration can be added. I have said that such individuals possess what I call a meaning disturbance as pathological play and that together with the splitting of mental contents there is also a defensively rigid denial of reality consideration in favor of destructive or grandiose and idealized illusion. One can understand how such an individual could welcome the opportunity offered by romantic-orgasmic experience to provide a physical "consummation" of grandiose, idealized, and exalted playful illusion about self and other. On the other hand, psychoneurosis, and also I think perversion, which is structured like fetishism, is characterized by a state of consciousness in which fantasy is "alienating . . . from reality" (Freud, 1911b, p. 218). Therefore, while such fantasy existence is experienced as not-real, it not only is structured so as to be indexed as not-real but also is experienced to be in conflict with reality. It is thus understandable how the natural, bio-psychological momentum which develops in the meaning apparatus for de-differentiation between real and not-real experience, in love-making, can be subject to intense conflict. What we often observe, of course, are the typical neurotic and perverse interferences with sexual function with which we are familiar, and this meaning apparatus perspective thus supplements our psychodynamic understanding about such psychopathology.

I turn again to some of Freud's (1920g) comments in *Beyond the Pleasure Principle.*

> Union with the living substance of a different individual increases . . . tensions introducing what might be described as fresh "vital differences" which then must be lived off. (p. 55)

And I want to cite again, but now more completely, certain comments from Freud's (1914c) Narcissism paper about love.

> A strong egoism is a protection against falling ill, but in the last resort we must begin to love in order not to fall ill, and we are bound to fall ill if, in consequence of frustration, we are unable to love. (p. 85)

If I attempt to understand these words from the viewpoint of meaning apparatus structure, function, and content, as I have used and developed this perspective in this investigation, I can say the following: Adult, clinical health includes good-enough, romantic love-making. Something which is eternal about the human condition is that love-making is a well; it rejuvenates human experience and behavior because it produces an unequalled, natural, playful infusion of grandiose, idealized, and exalted experience into the reality of one's adult life.

8

Conclusions and a Comment for Clinical Practice

I will summarize by stating certain conclusions which also will constitute my response to another question raised by Preyser (1975) about the concept of splitting. After this I will raise a treatment issue produced by the framework used in this paper.

Preyser's (1975) question: "Who or what is doing such splitting?" (p. 4) A thing (a what) does not do splitting. Only a person (a who) does anything, including splitting. To say that an ego splits is to confuse a useful, theoretical construct about a psychic system with a person. Actually, I here only repeat and agree with Preyser's (1975) own answer to the question he raises. But this same issue of reification applies to any of our psychic system terms. And I do not conclude from this that our theoretical comprehension of personality will be better off without the ideas of splitting and denial as I have used them in this investigation. These ideas of splitting and denial (disavowal) are now often used in our literature because they are responsive to important psychological realities we come upon in our work with various kinds of borderline, narcissistic, false-self, schizoid, etc., individuals.

But to use this idea of splitting in a theoretical context of the psychic system ego is a contradiction in terms. A clarifying theoretical context about this idea of splitting has to do with attributes of the self-construct prior to mature personality structuralization. We use the concept of an ego (psychic system), an id, together with the superego when a person's experience and behavior is conceptualized to possess a certain order of structural complexity. If such be the case, we then can conceptualize a (psychic system) ego in connection with a particular person, and we cannot use splitting in any way to characterize the functioning of such a substructure of personality. The ego (psychic system) indicates the achievement of certain procedures for the organization of meaning (consciousness) which, precisely, signal an emergence from other, immature procedures for meaning production which are defensively made use of in splitting and denial. Now, repression emerges as a basic defense (together with other defenses built upon it). Also, a new differentiation occurs between self and other, and the internalization of this new capability is the capacity for self-observation. This includes a new relationship and function for language as a symbolic vehicle. There also is the emergence of a new differentiation and integration with regard to real versus not-real experience. Now we can speak about a difference between neurotically or perversely conflicted fantasy versus reality, versus clinically healthy "imaginative living" (Winnicott, 1953, p. 14) which enriches existence indexed as real.

I have emphasized one reading of Freud's concepts of a life and death instinct to be a matter of how humans, like other reasonably complex life forms, are prefigured, given an expectable environment (Hartmann, 1939) to use psychic tension for an ontogenesis of psychic structure (life instinct), or to continuously repeat a pathological misuse of undeveloped psychic organization in an attempt to minimize or eliminate psychic tension (death instinct). I understand splitting and denial to express such a pathological "compulsion to repeat" (Freud, 1920g, p. 19) with regard to the functioning—indeed also the very content—of the meaning apparatus.

Altogether, I do not think Freud was even-handed in his treatment of not-real experience with respect to an ordinary person. But it is just this, a positive significance for not-real experience, which binds together the innovative, theoretical contributions of such as Winnicott (e.g., 1951, 1953, 1954b), Kohut (e.g., 1971, 1977), and Loewald (1975) about clinically healthy personality development, as well as the nature of the psychoanalytic process. Freud (e.g., 1908e, 1911b) had a deep appreciation, one might even say awe, for artists and the relevance of the work they produced for comprehension of reality, something I have termed paradoxical creation. But I think there also is no doubt that Freud (1911b) considered science to be in a class by itself with regard to the evaluation placed upon reality. I believe this is incorrect, and we deal here with matters of procedure rather than substance. To put this another way, psychoanalysis can appreciate better than it does the scientific objectives of art, and the art involved in the paradoxical creation known as scientific theory.[1] Obviously, Freud's genius enabled his imagination to find a lifetime of deep and full expression in the theoretical, paradoxical creation which characterizes science. But inasmuch as science possesses such paradoxical creation, it is not entirely correct to say that "science is no illusion" (Freud, 1927c, p. 56) of any sort.

I believe another correction is needed with regard to the place we accord not-real experience in the lives of those clinically healthy adults for whom imagination does not entail some kind of paradoxical creation. Freud (1924e) once actually stated that "neurotic fantasy is like the play of [presumably clinically healthy] children" (p. 187), and I think this is not correct. I have chosen to emphasize another insight of Freud's (1911b) concerning neurotic fantasy, and have made this the critical feature, namely, that neurotic fantasy is "alienating" (p. 218) in regard to reality because of conflict. I believe such a view actually is more consistent with Freud's own writing about childish play. Freud (1908e) understood full well the importance of play for the clinically healthy child and said this quite directly:

> A child's play is determined by wishes: in point of fact by a single wish—one that helps in his upbringing—to be big and grownup. (p. 146)

However, Freud (1908e) also had the opinion that the clinically healthy child distinguishes "quite well" (p. 144) between play and reality. But the work of Piaget (e.g., 1945) makes clear that the meaning apparatus of the young child does not possess properties that function so as to enable authentic differentiation between experience indexed as real versus not-real. This development is produced in part by a mature meaning apparatus which emerges in middle latency (Steingart, 1969), and then we can speak about clinically healthy "imaginative living" (Winnicott 1953, p. 14) which authentically differentiates and integrates between real and not-real experience, with the latter enriching the former. But the clinically healthy young child—precisely in part because what an experience means will be determined by some immediate, compelling attributes—has a high regard for what I have called actuality, and thus he or she will accommodate to changing circumstances adaptively. In this way, the play of the clinically healthy young child and the "imaginative living" of the like-minded adult show a functional similarity to each other.

I have used Winnicott's (1953) term "imaginative living" (p. 14) to create what I believe is a certain necessary theoretical and clinical distinction. On the one hand, there is conflicting neurotic or perverse fantasy which is "alienating" (Freud, 1911b, p. 218) from reality. On the other hand, there can be imaginative experience which also is understood and felt to be not-real representation differentiated from reality, but which serves only to enliven our involvement with reality and the "community of man" (Freud, 1912x, p. 74). I here take exception to Freud's (1908e) statement that "a happy person never fantasizes, only an unsatisfied one" (146). I point out again that Freud, in an extraordinary way because of his genius, had a continuous outlet for his imaginative capabilities in the realm of scientific paradoxical creation. An "honorable ancestor" of such not-real creation is located in Winnicott's (1953) idea of the "transitional object" (p. 1). I believe that the same considerations and characteristics I have described for clinically healthy play apply to this initial foray into not-real experience in the life cycle. We would expect a clinically healthy toddler, in a situation where some actuality (hunger, fear, etc.) becomes dominating, to foresake the transitional object in favor of the safety and satisfaction provided by the actual mother; if this is not the case, we already have evidence for a disturbed toddler.[2]

To these ideas of clinically healthy play, "imaginative living" (Winnicott, 1953, p. 14), and paradoxical creation, I have added the concept of gratifying (grandiose and idealizing) pathologically playful illusion, and indicate how I believe it characterizes especially what we have come to term narcissistic personality. I also have suggested that if what I have described as a meaning disturbance alternately or predominantly shows as painful pathological play, especially saturated with orally aggressive content, we tend toward a diagnosis of borderline personality. As important as I consider it to be to grant a place for a clinically healthy use of not-real experience in adult life, and see this as a functional continuation of clinically healthy childish play, it is just as important not to confuse what I have described as pathological play with such a clinically healthy integration of not-real experience. I have drawn an analogy between a meaning disturbance as pathological play and adult perversion. That is to say, pathological play is a "perversion" of reality considerations just as actual perversion represents a corruption of genital sexuality. I also have emphasized that such a meaning disturbance already can be evident and contrasted with healthy play in the young child. At whatever point in the life cycle we observe a meaning disturbance, its presence implicates the operations of splitting and denial which always are to be regarded as rigidified defensive operations which work against the general development of psychological organization, and in particular indicate psychopathological interference in progressive maturity of the meaning apparatus.

Any time from latency onward, one can observe an incredible disjointedness about meaning production. Individuals who plainly and pervasively employ splitting and denial also can demonstrate an adequate, or more usually, even superior thought capability outside a core self and object representation area which regulates self and object esteem and/or emotional survival. I believe this state of affairs is part and parcel of what Winnicott (1968) called "false self" (p. 140) development. With respect to a theory of development, there are at least three interrelated questions for future investigation. (1) What determines age expectable, overall growth in the representational apparatus, from "pictorial" (Freud, 1900a, p. 340) to more general (abstract or verbal) thought? (2) If we collect a "cross-section" at any period in early childhood about such core self and object representations which regulate self and object esteem or emotional survival, then there would be found a range of concepts: from representations which still center about impelling, pleasure/pain features to prototype images which center about different functional kinds of content. What determines how meaning production is distributed within this range? (3) What determines the chronic maintenance and (mis)use of immature meaning structure for splitting and denial? In any event, borderline, narcissistic, etc., pathology which involves what I have called a meaning disturbance should be distinguished from schizophrenic "fragmentation" (e.g., Kohut, 1971, p. 215; Jacobson 1957, p. 134) of ideas, which is the result of condensations and displacements (primary processes) acting upon such immature organizations of meaning (see, for example, Peto, 1964).[3]

I have taken this frame of reference and applied it to the question of the normal and abnormal development of love, hate, and ambivalence. I have insisted that love, even in the young child, includes an attachment to the actuality of the mother and father who protect and nurture. And I have also stressed that love, in its inception and throughout the life cycle, must involve not only object idealization but special, grandiose feeling attached to the self representation, as well as what I have called exaltation of the representation of the libidinal drive itself. With clinically normal personality development, and this includes the emergence of a mature meaning apparatus in a core area of self-object representation which regulates self and object esteem and/or emotional survival, these not-real imaginative constructions are understood and felt to be a source of symbolic enrichment differentiated from reality. I consider that, with love, what I have called an exaltation of sexuality occurs which we most directly and immediately experience as romance. This involves also transformation of a preemptory and periodic libidinal drive into a relatively continuous bio-social desire for a selected other person which we experience as longing. With sexuality which is romantic, there develops during love-making an impetus in the meaning apparatus toward a natural de-differentiation about real versus not-real grandiose, idealized, and exalted experience. Thus, romantic love is a never-ending source for a natural sublime experience which can enrich the reality of our lives. I do not believe that any of these characteristics of love can be handled by our customary concepts of libidinal sublimation, or some sort of idea of sexual drive inhibition, inasmuch as such concepts imply some curtailment in pleasurable aim or release which does not characterize the actual experience of romantic love. I also have indicated how a related set of ideas applies to the emergence of hate, which is thus to be contrasted to our customary concept of the aggressive drive.

Love, in its origin, is inherently dangerous because of a potential for destruction of the loved other as well as interference with an autonomous main-ten-ance of an individuated self representation. These inherent dynamic dangers which characterize love mark it as different from simple drive gratification involvement or attachment behavior. I believe that the concept of ambivalence should be reserved for the emergence of clinically normal love versus hate desires in the young child, and that a term like splitting-ambivalence be reserved for a pathological misuse of an immature meaning apparatus which rigidly defends against one or another of the dangers which inhere in love and hate. I am not certain whether some degree of defensive splitting-ambivalence is inevitable in early normal development. There is no current observation that convinces me that this must be the case. But I am convinced that splitting, theoretically, should be distinguished from the working of an immature but normal meaning apparatus which structures meaning into prototype-image representations, among which vivid, impelling qualities of love and hate experience certainly will be included. Inasmuch as development in the meaning apparatus is a necessary but insufficient condition for a structured integration of ambivalent experience, authentic self or object constancy cannot be said to exist prior to mid-latency (Steingart, 1969). With regard to adult psychopathology which shows splitting and denial, pathological maintenance of such an immature meaning apparatus makes self or object constancy impossible to achieve. The gradual regulation of ambivalent experience which one observes in the clinically healthy young child derives from a growing tolerance for ambivalence. In turn, this tolerance for ambivalence derives from the child's sense of his or her own increasing capability to determine loving or hating effects and so control the psychological space between himself or herself and the mother.

Once personality matures into id, ego, and superego psychic systems, not-real representation is now fully differentiated from experience indexed as real, and we can speak about ideals pertinent to the essential function of each of these psychic systems. I have described love as an id-related ideal of drive gratification and indicated how there are other ideals which can be related to the essential functions of the ego and superego psychic systems (Steingart, 1969).

I also have indicated how an individual's not-real experience may undergo another emergence, beyond ideal content which is concretely and thus securely related to the consistent presence of some particular reality matrix, and becomes what I have termed paradoxical creation. In part, this can occur because ideal representation—indeed all representation—now is not only differentiated from experience indexed as real but known to be humanly made (inventions). This means an individual can now experience himself or herself to be someone who creates meaning, which, paradoxically, illuminates a reality which is understood to possess no necessary, secure basis for such meaning. I have described certain features of (especially contemporary) religion, as well as the arts, science, and philosophy, and finally myth, and understood such features as paradoxical creations about the basic functions of, respectively, the psychic systems superego, ego, and id. But, as paradoxical creations, no such realization about our psychic system functioning can ever find a secure basis in any particular reality matrix. I have emphasized a second reading of Freud's (1920g) concepts of a life and death instinct to be mythological, paradoxical creations about the ultimate, instinctual, eternal reality a human being may possess about his or her physical existence.[4]

I will raise only one consideration about psychoanalytic practice. The consideration is not new—the issue of other-than-only-language activity in the treatment room (e.g., Ferenczi, 1931; Balint, 1968; Eissler, 1950, 1953)—but the framework used here offers a particular viewpoint. Psychoanalysis is a talking therapy. Of course, treatment experience must involve intense emotions and sensation if it is to be any good. But it remains true that language is the customary means by which we expect individuals being treated by psychoanalysis to communicate their experience to us, and by which we indicate to them our interpretative, empathic understanding of their experience. But we really mean more than just this act of communication, as important as this is. We believe that language, at a certain point in the life cycle, implicates a different order of knowing about one's existence (e.g., Piaget, 1945; Vygotsky, 1962), something Freud (1915e) once called "a higher psychical organization" (p. 202), and that this kind of comprehension is a necessary but insufficient condition for insight. However,

Piaget's (e.g., 1945) work makes clear that language does not exist as a differentiated symbolic vehicle for the young child who is not yet in possession of authentic class concepts. The young child thinks in terms of vivid, impelling, prototype images—and these images are more naturally realized in actions and drawings, together with sensations and perceptions produced by actions. Just this circumstance always has been recognized to exist in child analysis. I also have cited A. Freud's (1968) observation that what is natural for the young child is that "not thought or speech but motor actions are their legitimate media of expression and communication" (p. 169). What is added by Piaget's (e.g., 1945) work is, first, the importance of the conceptual differentiation between thought and speech (language) as a symbolic vehicle. Then these "motor actions" (A. Freud, 1968, p. 169) of a young child must indeed be understood to be the natural form of realization for the kinds of prototype-image representations of which a young child is capable.

But if I am correct, this is true not only of the young child, but also of borderline and narcissistic adults who predominantly employ splitting and denial, who possess a meaning disturbance and thus are not fully "into" their ideas with language. So there is, I believe, a special problem here for the psychoanalytic treatment of such adults (and children who are in latency or older). The psychoanalytic situation must provide not only awareness of dynamically unconscious motivation but also must provide for such individuals' insights into their equally defended-against, special, other-than-only-language organization of consciousness. A contention that all of this must always only be done with words amounts to an argument that it does not matter—for either actor or audience—whether a play is read or performed. But a play is created for performance, and in certain respects, so is the meaning organization of individuals who predominantly employ splitting and denial. Thus, such individuals who I describe as having a meaning disturbance need a psychoanalytic situation which will accept, at least for certain critical moments, other-than-only-language realizations of meaning. In one sense, this is a quite traditional idea. Is not lying on a couch, in addition to its dynamic and object relations aspects, an other-than-only-language, physical realization of meaning?

I am now in an area staked out by Eissler's (1953) important concept of a treatment parameter. Eissler states the following about this idea of a treatment parameter:

> I define the parameter of a technique as a deviation, both qualitative and quantitative, from the basic model technique, that is to say, from a technique which requires interpretation as the *exclusive* tool. (p. 110 italics mine)

But what is not clear, as Eissler (1953) also indicates, has to do with boundaries "beyond which therapeutic measures create an irreparable damage to the [interpretative] transference relationship" (p. 112). Actually, to continue with this metaphor of boundaries, this idea of a treatment parameter implicates the existence of some vast, so-to-speak, unexplored clinical practice territory, and a demarcation (conceptualization) of various states of meaning organization within this domain must be accomplished. Only then can we consider how any particular treatment parameter may facilitate or interfere with the development and productive resolution of the transference relationship. Treatment parameters actually cited by Eissler (e.g., 1950, 1953) possess at least two important differences: First, there is variation with respect to how concrete is the therapeutic activity (e.g., language versus giving money); second, there can be variability in terms of who initiates such activity into the treatment relationship.

It is not my intention here to consider fully these important questions. But I do want at least to indicate how a perspective about the meaning apparatus organization of the individual in treatment is relevant. Eissler (1950) indicates how "concreteness plays a greater role in the mental life of the child . . . [but also adds that such concreteness as adult psychopathology] is no index of . . . intellectual endowment" (p. 117). Now these comments by Eissler (1950) specifically come from a discussion about the psychoanalytic treatment of delinquents. But I believe they apply with equal force to that entire range of borderline, narcissistic, etc., individuals who possess what I have called a meaning disturbance which shows as pathological play. Indeed, such individuals do have a "tendency to accept only the concrete part of external reality as valid" (Eissler, 1950, p. 114). But this is not only a dynamically determined insistence upon some tangible libidinal or love gratification, or an attribute of some very early object relationship, although both of these are true. In addition, the prototype-image representation meaning apparatus of such individuals is such that any experience which touches upon a substantive matter of self and object esteem regulation and/or emotional survival *can only be known* through some such concrete activity and sensation. In other words, in addition to dynamic and object relationship reasons, this factor of such an actual immature meaning apparatus also serves to create a special treatment situation and issue.

Inasmuch as another characteristic of such an immature meaning-making apparatus is an insufficient differentiation between real and not-real construction, a special issue is created for what is real versus not-real experience in the treatment relationship. Grandiose, idealized, versus degraded, humiliated, etc., representations, for individuals who possess such a meaning disturbance, naturally will tend to be experienced as actual. This is an altogether different thing from our concept of transference. We mean by transference that productive maintenance of intense experience which is certainly felt as if real, but nevertheless remains essentially capable of insightful analysis from a realistic point of view (e.g., Loewald, 1975). This presupposes the existence of a representation-making apparatus which already possesses a differentiation between not-real experience (fantasy) and experience indexed as real. (In the case of the young child, the parallel capability would be a relatively free movement between play and actuality.) Therefore, one can say about the treatment for individuals who possess such a meaning disturbance that the problem is to create a productive transference relationship, whereas, with clinically neurotic individuals, treatment makes use of a transference relationship which issues out of an already existing differentiation between not-real experience (fantasy) and reality. There are two considerations with respect to treatment parameters which, in my experience, tend to so facilitate the creation of such a productive transference experience. First, any concrete activity which is introduced and accepted into the treatment relationship is best introduced by the analysand and not by the therapist. Second, whatever concrete activity is introduced and accepted into the treatment relationship is to be regarded as material for immediate or eventual verbal interpretation.

I will not here examine in any great detail the relationship between such an opportunity for other-than-only-language realization of meaning and various connotations of the concept of "acting out" (see, for example, A. Freud, 1968). I do believe that at least some of what we observe as acting out that is destructive to an analysis occurs just because the psychoanalytic relationship will not accept instances of such other-than-only-language realization of meaning for borderline, narcissistic, etc., individuals who possess what I have termed a meaning disturbance.

I do not think what I here describe as a possible necessity for other-than-only-language realization of meaning is the same as what Freud (1905e) meant by "acting out" in his case of Dora. With Dora, Freud believed he was dealing with neurotic personality organization. This means that language has achieved a certain kind of analyst-analysand compatability—one could say a certain status. Language, now, is not just a suitable vehicle for communication but a completely satisfactory basis for the realization of meaning in a human relationship. The analyst's verbal interpretation is directed to an analysand whose consciousness can be organized with meaning structures, which, themselves, already have achieved a language-compatible autonomy from "perceptions [to be read all manner of diverse, impelling, prototype representation qualities] which bring . . . knowledge" (Freud, 1940a, p. 204). This kind of organization of consciousness is not present in a core area of an object representation for individuals who possess what I have called a meaning disturbance, even though such people may well be not just verbally facile but intriguing and brilliant individuals. This perspective in no way mitigates the importance of verbal interpretation by the analyst, either in general, and particularly interpretation directed toward dynamically unconscious psychosexual and aggressive drive conflict. Quite the opposite is the case. If anything, it is even more critical for the analyst to be a model for linguistically organized experience for individuals who possess a meaning disturbance, and which can include such instances for a felt necessity for an other-than-only-language realization and meaning. This is accomplished by the analyst's steadfast functioning as a verbal interpreter of everything which transpires in the psychoanalytic relationship, including (at an appropriate time) verbal interpretation of such other-than-only-language realization of meaning. An instance of such other-than-only-language realization of meaning is exactly what I have in mind about the inherently playful nature of a meaning disturbance. Such an instance is part and parcel of splitting and denial, and therefore in an intimate—albeit defensive—relationship to dynamically unconscious conflict. Put another way, each aspect of what I have described as a meaning disturbance is something which is dynamically and unconsciously produced, the awareness of which is subject to resistance and requires (sooner or later) verbal interpretation made to an individual who is able to use such interpretation for analysis.

Should, then, what I describe as a meaning disturbance be conceived of as a "developmental arrest" (Stolorow and Lachmann, 1980, p. 5)? If what is meant by a "developmental arrest" is some psychological immaturity, considered clinically healthy at one point in the life cycle, and now (to me mysteriously) maintained but not because the behavior or experience in question intimately, continuously subserves dynamic conflict, then everything I have conceived about a meaning disorder surely is unlike any idea of some such simple, direct arrest in development. Indeed, given a neurologically intact child or adult, I would not apply such an idea of "developmental arrest" (Stolorow and Lachmann, 1980, p. 5) to the maintenance of any psychic immaturity, and I consider that this concept itself perches precariously upon a vision of therapy as a kind of benevolent parentalism.

I want now to present some brief clinical material which illustrates these ideas. A young woman in treatment employed massive splitting and denial (with playful illusion) in order to avoid experiencing a profound splitting-ambivalence conflict with me. She harbored enormous hate as well as love toward me. But this was directly evident only in two kinds of very occasional, conscious thoughts. First, she could have the thought that my "penis is on fire," and second, that a pipe pick, almost always in view, was pushed into the opening of my penis. She always became quite anxious and humiliated by such thoughts, which she understood to be completely irrational, and any attempt I made to discuss why such thoughts would occur was vigorously resisted. She simply refused to discuss it. Treatment at this time almost exclusively was sitting up, and this had been her choice. She expressed anxiety about how overwhelmingly disorganized she expected she would become if she were lying down on the couch. Also, she said that for her to even think about lying on the couch produced a feeling of such intense humiliation and degradation that she could not "submit" herself to it.

One day this young woman announced as she walked into the room that she wanted to sit on my desk while she talked. I did not feel it would be correct to object, but asked if she had any idea why she wanted to do this. She responded immediately, with no smile or any other expression which might indicate embarrassment, "Then I'll be bigger than you." The patient then described an experience which she later said would have felt too humiliating to talk about without benefit of the change in physical relationship between us. We then discussed the experience itself, which involved the loss of her own viewpoint (self representation) in the physical presence of her mother, and her use of this playful illusionary rearrangement of our bodies to avoid intense humiliation. She wanted to believe she was bigger than I by physically elevating her body in relationship to mine. There was, incidentally, a good deal of evidence about an extremely intrusive as well as overstimulating father who would often "ride" this young woman as a young child on his back with her legs clasped about his neck. There is some reason to believe that she experienced frequent orgasm in this way. She could not recall any incident throughout her entire life of a self-initiated intention to masturbate.

It is my experience that such a treatment moment, while not necessarily frequent, can have a special importance. Certainly this importance can be stated in terms of a dynamic or object relationship aspect of the experience. But I believe what is equally cogent, and what makes the episode so critical, is the acceptance of a meaning structure as it really is organized at the moment in the psychic apparatus, for purposes of analysis. Once this occurs, I believe dynamic and object relationship aspects of such meaning are able to be present in a way that can enhance the creation of productive transference experience. The immediate or eventual verbal interpretation by the therapist of such a critical moment ideally may then produce verbal exchange which facilitates "a higher psychical organization" (Freud, 1915e, p. 202). Such verbalization which follows upon acceptance of such a critical moment of a physical realization of meaning has a better chance not to be experienced as an intrusion made by the therapist, which only will repeat basic trauma.

And what is this basic trauma? It is, of course, complex, including instinctual drive dynamics, as well as matters pertinent to object relationship and narcissistic psychopathology. The perspective developed in this investigation emphasizes another aspect of this complex, theoretical scenario: That there is a vital matter of the construction of a differentiation between experiences indexed as real (actual in the young child) and as not-real. That clinical health involves not simply such a differentiation but also an enriching, patterned interplay between the not-real and real (actual) experience. That without such a relatively conflict-free integration of real (actual) versus not-real, neither our drives nor our desires can be psychologically viable, and consequently we cannot experience ourselves as substantive. That individuals who possess what I have described as a playful meaning disturbance rigidly maintain belief in not-real experience in a core area of self and object representation which governs self and object regulations and/or survival; and that such belief is about both aggressively psychically painful and libidinally psychically pleasurable mental content. That while such a meaning disturbance (splitting and denial) leaves linguistic programs intact, what can be experienced as critical for this core area of self and object representation is a playful, other-than-only-language realization of meaning. That in all of this language competence and performance is not the seed of clinical health or psychopathology, but the fruit.[5] That the seed has to do with the emergence of the individual as someone who makes meaning both real (actual in the young child) and not-real.

What do we understand to be happening when a young child who has just emerged as a maker-of-meaning, now is working out the representation of himself or herself as someone who produces stool for the mother? Certainly we have learned from Freud (e.g., 1908b) that a child will represent the instinctual drive conflicts which inhere in this experience. And we have come to understand the profound implications of toilet training for the child's representation of himself or herself as someone who is autonomous (Erikson, 1950), individuated (e.g., Mahler, Pine, and Bergman, 1975), and who makes a clinically healthy, self-enhancing, grandiose stool gift to an idealized mother (Kohut, e.g., 1977). But in all of this, and yet still a separate matter from all of this, is the issue of the child as a maker-of-meaning about these diverse aspects of the toilet-training experience. Psychopathology can involve acknowledgement of the child as a maker of such meanings but reject the meanings so made. Or, what is still worse, there can be a negation of the child altogether as the originator of any meaning. The occurrence of the latter is the condition which is necessary if the individual is to acquire a meaning disturbance. Such an individual especially could come to feel that some playful, other-than-only-language realization of meaning is a necessity in order to experience himself or herself as a vital originator of meaning.

Descartes's (1637) famous solution to a well-known philosophical conun--drum was, "I think; therefore I am" (p. 221). What I am saying is that this is not just a philosophical question. It is a critical matter which arises in human development at a point in the life cycle when the child emerges as a maker-of-meaning. That what is as subtle as it is significant for the young child, who now has awareness of meaning, is whether conditions produce the sense that it is he or she who originates meaning—"*I* think; therefore *I* am." (Descartes 1637, italics mine.)[6]

Notes

CHAPTER 2

On Splitting and the Psychoanalytic Concept of Development

1. I have indicated how I believe the idea of development is inconceivable without some sort of ideas about progressive differentiation and integration which produce emergent structure(s), and which thus demonstrate emergent function and (at least in humans) content. I now have added that development also will show, nevertheless, possession of historical continuity (connection). A well-known example of all of this in animal learning research involves Harlow's (1949) demonstration that a monkey can be taught so as to acquire a "learning set . . . learning how to learn" (p. 51). Once established, this set or strategy enables the monkey to solve any presented, novel discrimination problem with only one trial, whereas previously, many trials would be necessary for a solution. Thus, an emergent structure is in evidence. But it is also clear that the establishment of this emergent organization is accomplished only through a gradual, continuous learning (developmental) process. Harlow (1949) states: "If such phenomena [i.e., learning sets] appear independently of a gradual learning history, we have not found them in the primate order." (p. 65)

I am not knowledgeable enough to state where one can say such development begins as a phenomenon in the evolution of complex animal life forms, or whether it characterizes even large-scale plant life.

If I understand anything about Whitehead's (1925) philosophical doctrine of "organism" (p. 38), he would attribute such life-like developmental attributes to inanimate nature as well. This is not only interesting but diametrically opposite to Freud's (1920g) application of the concept of a death instinct to animate nature, which I will discuss shortly. It is also interesting to realize that these two men were writing such different formulations at about the same time.

2. Kohut (1977) appeals to a "principle of complementarity" (p. xv) which enables us to view the self as something other than mental content, and also see it "in a broader sense . . . that puts the self in the center" (p. xv). In this connection, Kohut (1977) states the following:

> We must learn to think alternatively, or even simultaneously, in terms of two theoretical frameworks; that we must, in accordance with a psychological principle of complementarity, recognize that a grasp of the phenomena encountered in our clinical work . . . requires two approaches: a psychology in which the self is seen as the center

> of the psychological universe, and a psychology in which the self is seen as a content of a mental apparatus. (p. xv)

With respect to this principle of complementarity, Kohut (1977) makes reference to a paper by Edelheit (1976). But the thrust of Edelheit's (1976) paper is not really about a psychological principle but a philosophical position as to how to approach the mind-body problem, as follows:

> When considering two complementary hypotheses, what is proper to the mode of discourse of one hypothesis is to be kept conceptually isolated from the context of the other. Specifically, one must avoid carrying over a neuro-physiological explanation into the exposition of psychological process, or vice versa. (p. 23)
>
> Essentially, the principle of complementarity is a rule for the use of language. (p. 28)

It is true that there have existed in physics complementary theories, such as the wave and corpuscular theories of light, in order to explain all of light's characteristics. But it is hardly true that physicists (see, for example, Toulmin and Goodfield, 1962), or philosophers of science (see, for example, Whitehead, 1925), have remained content with such a view of nature. In any event, I beleive the application of such a principle of complementarity to this matter of self versus psychic system theory is a big and unnecessary jump.

Modell's (1975) contention that the concepts of self representation versus object representation are not on the same conceptual footing is not something with which I can agree because, as he states it, no distinction is made between structure and both self representation and object representation content which is produced by such structure. Thus, I would say psychic structure is not on the same conceptual footing as either self or object representation content. It will be understood that when I use the term self or object representation in this investigation, I always have in mind the operation of such psychic structure, and I simply want to focus upon qualities in mental content.

3. Piaget (1968) understands this as the acquisition of a basic qualitative identity which is the basis for all later development of symbolic intelligence. I am indebted to Dr. K. Oran for making known to me research by Anthony (e.g., 1958) in this area which illustrates such cognitive insufficiency. Rappaport's (1957b) statement, "Drive organization is conceptual, too, in the broad sense in which conceptual organization means equivalence organization" (p. 633), certainly is the same idea.

4. One can find in our literature language like a "drive toward individuation" (Mahler, 1975, p. 9), and perhaps a term like "drive" is selected because of Freud's (1920g) use of the term "life instincts" (p. 40) in connection with the phenomenon of development. But if we use a word like "drive" in this context, we would have to go on to say a human has a "drive" to acquire "drives" (among other things). I believe the two phenomena to which the term "drive" alludes (development and motivation) are so different that the same term should not be used.

CHAPTER 3
The Emergence and Growth of a Meaning Apparatus

1. Or, to use another metaphor, it would be as if the identity of all the actually diverse men and women who exist were referable only to a select few preconcept, prototype, image-representation "movie stars" of meaning. Thus, a particular man would be known as (mean) Gary Cooper because of some impelling perceptual-like quality, say, tall gauntness. Another man would be (mean) Charles Laughton because of large jowels. But the first man could suddenly become (mean) James Stewart if he began to speak with a nasal twang, and this perceptual quality became predominating. Thus, no actually consistent human being would retain stable identity (meaning), and neither could there exist a stable class concept (stable attribution of a particular movie star identity).

The fact that certain religions (e.g., Hebrew and Moslem) prohibit images of the deity may be relevant to this "magical" phenomenon of immature, prototype, image representation.

2. I use the word "makes" quite deliberately. The fact that a young child begins to learn how to make meaning at a time which at least roughly corresponds to the same developmental period in which the toddler learns to "make" stool has profound significance. I believe that all of the important narcissistic, drive, dynamic, and object relationship issues which we have come to understand in connection with this anal period carry over to the "making" of ideas. There is a connection here to the work of Bion (e.g., 1954), but a further, detailed examination of this is beyond the scope of this investigation. Werner and Kaplan (1963) provide useful, illustrative material as regards such immature cognitive functioning.

Piaget (1945) acknowledges borrowing this term "participation" from Levi-Bruhl's (e.g., 1928) important studies of pre-literate cultures. One example among the many cited relates to our North American Indian, and how the Indian believed that the taking of the scalp conferred permanent power to the possessor over the slain enemy.

3. We have in our language the expression, "He or she knows which side of the bread is buttered," which I think captures the sense of what I mean about how a clinically healthy young child is supremely responsive to "actualities."

CHAPTER 4
On the Concept of a Meaning Disturbance—Pathological Play

1. A bright, quite verbal little girl, close to two years old, was asked to answer, "What is a Mommy?" with her mother not present. Among her answers were:

> Mommy a take-care-of-me. Mommy has two eyes and two ears. Mommy a person. Mommy go play tennis . . . come home and play with me.

We have in our language the saying, "Seeing is believing," which, I think, relates to this state of affairs. But we should understand that "seeing" here does not refer to hallucination but to how a preconcept always is organized as a prototype image-representation which always is "centered" (Piaget, e.g., 1945, p. 235) about some impelling perceptual-like qualities for meaning.

2. Lichtenberg and Slap (1973) state that their use of the concept of splitting to describe the normal way in which mental contents are organized in early childhood is in keeping with Hartmann's (1947) construct of an "organizing function" (p. 62). I do not agree. Hartmann (1947) did describe such an "organizing function," but he carefully indicated how this organizing function "develops only gradually, parallel to the development of the ego, . . . [and] it partly replaces more primitive regulations" (p. 62). Actually, Hartmann (1947), in his paper, proposes the term "organizing function" to replace Nunberg's (1930) concept of a synthetic function "because in the concept of organization we include elements of differentiation as well as of integration" (p. 62). Thus, Hartmann here emphasizes how developmental processes of differentiation and integration characterize the life cycle, but, at different points in development, such differentiation and integration show emergent properties. The perspective of this investigation thus agrees with Hartmann's suggestion that the concept of a synthetic function (as emergent integrative and differentiating processes) be reserved theoretically to tally with the advent of the psychic system ego. Further, there is nothing in Hartmann's (1947) paper which suggests that splitting be construed as a normal "primitive regulation." As far as I am aware, Hartmann never said this.

3. I believe that comments made in the previous footnote (2) also are relevant to this point.

Chapter 5

A Comparative Psychopathology Approach to Splitting and Denial

1. This point still holds even if free associations had been the special means of recovering into consciousness the defended-against experience.

2. It is possible that the extent to which verbal or visual material contributes as a day residue for dream production is also (perhaps inversely) related to this matter of a visual versus verbal organization of consciousness.

3. The maintenance in the literature of Freud's viewpoint about the relationship between denial and reality, taken together with the realization that denial has to do with all manner of perceptual-like quality, has led to statements like the following:

> When the instinct representations have become conscious and make a claim on the ego to be accepted as reality (which would be called here "internal reality", but which can be treated by the ego as if external), denial may make its appearance. (Lewin, 1961, p. 53)

> We recall that originally the child cannot distinguish between external and internal reality . . . If denial handles psychic manifestations as though they were external reality, the prerequisite for denial of the inner world must be a partial regression—not to this earliest but to a "concretistic" infantile stage where the child,though already aware of the difference between internal and external world, between himself and objects, still treats both in the same manner. (Jacobson, 1957, p. 125)

I believe such statements are unnecessarily complicated, as well as at least potentially confusing. At first it is suggested than an individual who uses denial is confusing something which is internal (an idea or a feeling) with something external (a perception), but then it is said that this is not the case. I believe one can state this differently, and more simply, in terms of the meaning apparatus perspective of this investigation. Denial in part occurs because the only way an immature mental apparatus can organize the meaning of what is objectively an internal experience (an idea or a feeling) is in terms of impelling, sensorial and/or motor qualities which inhere in an experience which is concrete and tangible. This does not have to do with any confusion between experience indexed as external and as internal. But an internal experience, like a feeling, can only be known by some such concrete, tangible relatedness to the external world.

There is also an issue here about a metaphysics congenial to psychoanalysis as a dynamic theory about human behavior and experience. But examination of this is beyond the scope of this investigation. I can, however, at least mention an interesting article by Novey (1955a) in this connection.

4. Dorpat (1979) apparently does the very same thing with the concept of denial. For example, Dorpat (1979) uses the concept of denial to describe an analysand's "first becoming aware of . . . his need to defend himself against angry feelings" (p. 106) in the second year of analysis. I believe this is more clearly conceptualized as the defense analysis of a repression.

5. This idea of playful, gratifying illusion adds a specific note to Moore's (1981) recent questioning about the "degree of gratification" (p. 250) provided narcissistic individuals by psychoanalysts who practice with Kohut's approach (see, for example,Goldberg, 1978).

6. McDougall (1980) uses the term illusion to depict fetishism and other perversions structured like fetishism. But I think it is clear that there is no difference between McDougall and myself with regard to either the phenomenology or the psychological organization of fetishism. But with this term illusion, McDougall intends to refer not only to the fetishist's conscious organization of fantasy (which she points out can often be quite barren like that of certain hysterics) but also to the fetishist's dynamically unconscious, fantastic, not-real beliefs about self and object representation. I use a term like playful illusion to include consciously held, gratifying, grandiose and idealizing not-real belief (which is nevertheless not schizophrenic reconstruction of reality), especially characteristic of the narcissistic personality disorder.

Also, when I speak about "perversions structured like fetishism," I have in mind a strict adherence to different kinds of psychological organization. Perverse, excitement at the sight of fire, for example, so that an actual nonsexual object, fire, is now dynamically associated with some unconscious sexual fantasy, is in this view similar to fetishistic construction. But we also have phenomena such as overt sado-masochism, male transvesticism, etc.; here, actual, sexual graficiation occurs within pathologically playful enactments of conscious, illusionary, not-real experience, in which one is omnipotent, a slave, a woman, and so forth. Still, while such sado-masochistic or transvestite enactments are not structured like fetishism, neither are they schizophrenic, hallucinatory, or delusional reconstruction of reality. Such enactments can occur in an individual who is schizophrenic (see, for example, Bach and Schwartz, 1972), but they are not, in themselves, examples of schizophrenic reconstruction. If anything, all else being equal, I would think such enactments work against necessity for a schizophrenic reconstruction of reality (see McDougall, 1980).

Later, in a comment for clinical practice, I will discuss and illustrate how an analysand can experience a necessity for an other-than-only-language realization of meaning in the analytic situation. But I believe what I later will describe as an other-than-only-language realization of meaning is analyzable and also importantly different from what I here describe as a perverse, conscious, not-real experience which includes actual sexual gratification.

7. Hanly and Masson (1976) also point out that what would follow from a strict reading of Kohut's (e.g., 1971, 1977) theory is that pathological narcissism could occur with clinically healthy object relations, and clinically this is not the case.

CHAPTER 6

On Real and Not-Real Meaning in Love, Hate, and Ambivalence

1. What I am saying is that, initially, in terms of a theory of meaning, the transitional object at first only has the status of a signal. This is similar to the way a green light is a signal to a driver that he or she can resume driving.

As far as I am aware, Winnicott never explicitly tied together in this way his formulations about the transitional object (Winnicott, 1953), and these comments I have cited about a "new kind of need" (Winnicott, 1954a, p. 267)—which I interpret as love desire. But if not, it certainly is implied in an additional comment I will now cite: "A new kind of need has arisen based on impulse . . . [and] the acceptance of ideas and of fantasy related to fact but not to be confused with fact" (Winnicott, 1954a, p. 267). I already have indicated why, instead of the terms "fantasy" versus "fact," I believe terms like not-real play versus actuality are more suited to the actual characteristics of the young child's meaning apparatus.

2. How, further, can we understand, in psychic energy terms, the way in which, in clinically healthy love, there naturally co-occurs self-enhancing grandiosity together with object idealization? Freud's (1914c) answer was as follows:

> Loving in itself, insofar as it involves longing and deprivation, lowers self-regard; whereas being loved, having one's love returned, and possessing the loved object, raises

> it once more. When libido is repressed, the erotic cathexis is felt as a severe depletion of the ego, the satisfaction of love is impossible, and the re-enrichment of the ego can be effected only by a withdrawal of libido from its objects. (pp. 99–100)

The closed-system finite model of psychic energy described here has been subject to much criticism (e.g., Panel, 1963). Notwithstanding this, it is important to stress, and I believe not generally appreciated, that Freud (1914c) certainly understood that the experience of a mutual, clinically healthy love, naturally, phenomenologically, brings an enhanced status of "enrichment" to both self and other.

Also, Kohut's (1971) statement "that narcissism follows an independent line of development" (p. 6)—as if the conception Freud (1941c) left us is in no way congruent with this idea—is, I think, not correct. Freud (1914c) stated the following:

> One part of self-regard is primary—the residue of infantile narcissism; another part arises out of the omnipotence which is corroborated by experience (the fulfillment of the ego ideal), while a third part proceeds from the satisfaction of object libido. (p. 100)

While I believe it is Kohut's contribution to describe a development of this "residue of infantile narcissism," there is nothing in this statement by Freud which makes such a development in this primary narcissism a difficulty for our theory. And neither should such a theory about the development of narcissism treat narcissism as unrelated to object love. In fact, I believe just the opposite is the case, and I will indicate how in a moment.

3. But if any of this is true, what does this imply for the importance of love in a modern society, physically "safe" in nature, faced with the problem of overpopulation in relation to dwindling resources?

4. It is worth noting that Mahler (e.g., 1968) herself, to whom we owe this emphasis on the term symbiosis, distinguishes this matter of development versus libidinal drive in statements like the following:

> [A patient] was forever searching for the "good" need-satisfying mother of his symbiotic phase. Yet at the same time he dreaded re-engulfment in symbiosis. As soon as he found an object, he arranged somehow to lose her, out of fear that she would engulf him and that he would thus "lose himself." (pp. 28–29)

5. While I have used important literature by Winnicott (1954) to understand the emergence of love, I do believe that Winnicott was off in his estimate of the developmental timing of this crucial event. Winnicott (1954) intuitively connected this achievement "at about five months" (p. 263) when the game of dropping things starts. But Piaget's work (e.g., 1951) indicates that authentic self versus object representation, which I take to be a necessary but insufficient condition for the emergence of love, will not occur until one to one-and-a-half years of age. Winnicott (1954) refers to Freud's (1920a) observation about a hide-and-seek game played by a child, but actually Freud here was describing an 18-month-old toddler (see also

Brody, 1980). Freud (1915b) once said the following about love, something which certainly emphasizes it as a developmental achievement.

> The transformation of "bad" instincts is brought about by two factors working in the same direction, an internal and an external one. The internal factor consists in the influence exercised on the bad (let us say the egoistic) instincts by eroticism—that is the human need for love, taken in its broadest sense. By the admixture of *erotic* components the egoistic instincts are transformed into *social* ones. *We learn to value being loved* as an advantage for which we are willing to sacrifice other advantages. The external factor is the force exercised by upbringing, which represents the claims of our cultural environment, and this is continued later by the direct pressure of that environment. Civilization has been attained through the renunciation of instinctual satisfaction . . . (p. 282, last italics mine).

What is interesting to realize is that Freudian theory has tended to be identified exclusively with the "external factor," i.e., with this idea of civilization as an antagonistic force against the instincts. But Freud also clearly describes here an "internal factor" which has to do with the emergence of love (and see also Freud, 1930a). This, I believe, tallies with literature I already have cited by Winnicott (1954a), and is congruent with research findings reported by Ainsworth and her colleagues (e.g., Stayton, Hogan, Ainsworth, and Salter, 1971).

Swinburne (1866), in a poem entitled "Dolores," soberly described the difference between romantic love and simple sexuality as follows:

> For the crown of our life as it closes
> Is darkness, the fruit thereof of dust;
> No thorns go as deep as roses
> And love is more cruel than lust. (289)

Freud (1921c) once, in a post-script to the Group Psychology Monograph, talked about how it can be that "A love relation gives place entirely to the sensual. . . . But at that point a regression has taken place to an early stage in sexual relations" (p.140).

6. There is also the matter of how emergent change(s) (development) with respect to the instinctual drives will contribute to variated loving and hating. This connects with Erikson's (1950) important conceptualization about libidinal zones and modes. It is beyond the scope of this investigation to pursue this further.

7. Does any other animal species possess love? Perhaps the answer to this question is to ask for the answer to another question: Does any other species show such negativism and ambivalence between offspring and mother?

8. There is a connection here to the work of Bion (e.g., 1954), but I will not pursue this further.

9. Consider the following from the Old Testament, and consider in what follows that "sins" means pathologically split mental contents: "For all sins love cures" (Proverbs, 10:12). The interesting thing is that the Bible does not say that "guilt cures" but that "love cures." I am grateful to Dr. L. Dimotrovsky for locating for me the source of the biblical literature.

Still other religious literature which I now can interpretatively consider has to do with the fabulous tale of Adam and Eve living nakedly in Paradise. From the point of view of the perspective developed in this investigation, so-called Paradise can be considered to be the maintenance of pathologically playful not-real experience. Reality knowledge, i.e., eating the apple, will always be not just in conflict with such pathological illusion, but completely unintegratable and hence the expulsion from Paradise. I have described the kind of romantic love which represents a clinically healthy integration of real and not-real experience.

But now, also from this point of view, the issue of public nudity (on beaches, etc.) does not become a serious psychological matter on moral or even strictly aesthetic grounds. The important question is this: Is public nudity an impediment to the maintenance of the not-real aspects of romantic love? But then, if it is, what does this say about a society which enables such a practice which works against romantic love?

10. We have in our language the expression, "Don't look a gift horse in the mouth," which I believe is related to this critical event.

11. We have in our langage the expression, "So-and-so bites the hand that feeds him or her," which I believe is related to this critical event.

12. Kohut's (e.g., 1971) concept of a "transmuting internalization" (p. 50) obviously represents a boundary-setting achievement with respect to self-esteem regulation for the young child. Once again, some important conceptualization by Erikson (e.g., 1950) ties in here with respect to his concept of identity, which represents still another boundary-setting achievement in the overall development of individuation.

I have already indicated that I believe it best to reserve the term identity only for emergent change in the psychic content of identificatory structures at adolescence. Erikson (1950) attempts to use this same term, identity, at least to allude to a continuous history of such representational content which I think is better left to the concept of individuation. Kohut (e.g., 1971, 1977) does an analogous thing in his use of the concept of self. I do not accept Kohut's (1971) contention that Erikson's (1950) identity concept is somehow not related to "depth psychology" (p. xiv). These two theorists simply are touching upon different aspects—matters of drive dynamics versus narcissistic dynamics—as they determine individuation throughout the life cycle.

CHAPTER 7

Further Development of Real and Not-Real Meaning in the Individual and Social Ideology—Paradoxical Creation

1. With respect to adolescence, the contribution of this further emergence of the meaning apparatus can be radical in other ways, and I will begin to describe some of these effects in a moment.

There is something else about the conception of love developed thus far in this investigation. I have made the centerpiece of this conception romantic love—romance—which certainly carries forward libidinal gratification, although now with a changed, emergent, elevated status for the gratification experience itself, self, and other. Passion is an eruption of libidinal excitement and longing, an acute state of extraordinarily intense, libidinal arousal. But still, I believe that passion also is exalted experience, and so, passion only can be the product of a relatively continuous state of romance. Passion also is not simply libidinal drive gratification.

Also, can love have psychological validity without erotic foundation? Such a question and answer is the subject matter of D. H. Lawrence's (1928) novel, *Lady Chatterley's Lover*. But what about the existence of love in a context wherein there is a natural decline of an erotic substrate? What about love in the extremely aged? What about the normal progression of parental love for children? I have no direct knowlege about love between extremely aged individuals, and observations about this are hard to obtain. However, it is interesting to realize that both these kinds of love do share a common characteristic. Both start with an erotic foundation—physical affection between young child and parent (hugging, kissing, etc.) certainly is natural and healthy—and there is a natural (relative) decline of this sensuous foundation. It seems reasonable to suppose, then, that love can further develop in a relative autonomy from such an initial, necessary, erotic substrate.

2. Therefore, for example, the death of a parent can produce an extraordinary but natural disillusionment for even a clinically healthy older child.

3. Note that I say "can," not that it must happen. I believe we take this to be at least a necessary, critical event for adolescence in a modern society, even if not sustained for most individuals.

4. At this point it should be clear that I have taken Winnicott's (1953) concept of "imaginative living" (p. 14) and created differentiations within this idea according to how the meaning apparatus functions at different periods of the life cycle.

5. Nowhere have I read a more graphic and dramatic description of science as paradoxical creation that these comments by Whitehead (1925):

> It was my good fortune to be present at the meeting of the Royal Society in London when the Astronomer Royal for England announced that . . . photographic plates . . . measured by his colleagues in Greenwich Observatory had verified the prediction of Einstein that rays of light are bent as they pass in the neighborhood of the sun. The whole atmosphere of tense interest was that of a Greek drama: We were the chorus commenting on the decree of destiny as disclosed in the development of a supreme incident. There was dramatic quality in the very staging—the traditional ceremonial, and in the background the picture of Newton to remind us that the greatest of scientific generalizations was now, after more than two centuries, to receive its first modification. (p. 11)

It is incorrect to believe that the arts, philosophy, and religion contain no sort of "corrective." Rather, these disciplines contain correctives which simply are unlike science. How else could we explain changing *movements* in these fields (not simply the work of one individual)?

6. The terminology I have adopted for this investigation would lead to the use of the

term paradoxical creation rather than illusion. The quotation used by Freud is from Schiller, and I have used the translation which appears in the Standard Edition.

7. Thus I would not, if I understand Loewald (1978) correctly, apply as he does the term "religious" (p. 77) to this entire, variated mental content which can be the subject matter for such a contemplative sense of eternality about the human condition.

How does myth accomplish this? Some comments made by Eissler (1958) about scriptural text probably apply to myth in general: "any attempt to cleanse the text [myth] of its contradictions or to reconcile it half-way with the requirements of logical or scientific thinking loosens its grip on the human mind" (p. 238). I suspect that not only content but also matters pertinent to sentence construction, or sequences of sentence construction (discourse) play a role in the emotional impact of myth. It may be that a system for the assessment of language behavior I developed and used in various research projects with Doctors Norbert Freedman and Stanley Grand at Downstate Medical Center would turn out to be relevant (Steingart, e.g., 1972, 1977).

8. I want to express my gratitude to Professors G. S. Schwartz and N. B. Arthur for their guidance into pertinent literature related to this topic.

Chapter 8

Conclusions and a Comment for Clinical Practice

1. Edman (1928) puts it this way:

> The human consciousness has always been uneasily curious as to what was really real. Now the nature of truth is a logical inquiry; the inquiry into nature of reality may very likely turn out to be primarily an aesthetic enterprise. Truth is always propositional; it is a statement about fact. But facts are data of immediate experience, and it is the special privilege of the fine arts to reveal immediate data with a clarity, intensity, and purity that promotes them as it were to a special degree of reality. (p. 52)

I always have been charmed, and impressed, by how Freud took note on one occasion of this matter of paradoxical creation in science. At the very end of that incredible, theoretical, tour de force, The Unconscious, Freud (1915e) sardonically used his just created theory against himself and had this to say about what he had just written:

> When we think in abstractions there is a danger that we may neglect the relations of words to unconscious thing-presentations, and it must be confessed that the expression and content of our philosophizing then begins to acquire an unwelcome resemblance to the mode of operation of schizophrenics. (p. 204)

2. Sperling (1963) has criticized Winnicott's concept of the transitional object with respect to this issue. But I think it is clear that Winnicott understood the difference between a clinically healthy and a pathological transitional object. There is, for example, Winnicott's (1953) illustration of the "string" (p. 15) as a pathological transitional object.

3. But it is true that Freud, at least at times, used these concepts of displacement and condensation to allude to normal, albeit immature childish thought, and I believe this has been a source of confusion. For example, Freud (1900a) once said, "When I described one of the psychical processes occurring in the mental apparatus as the "primary" one what I had in mind was not merely considerations of relative importance and efficiency; I intended also . . . chronological priority." (p. 603)

4. Altogether then, I have considered Freud's life and death instinct concepts as a kind of manifest content, to which I have given two interpretations as a kind of latent meaning.

5. Looming, we might even say lurking, behind this entire investigation is the question of language, i.e., the place of language in psychoanalytic theory and practice. This complex question requires its own investigation.

6. In a fascinating speculation about Descartes's philosophy from the viewpoint of personal trauma, Eisenbud (1978) points out that this philosopher suffered the loss of his mother at thirteen months. Descartes's mother actually died in sibling childbirth, a fact which the philosopher denied throughout his life, according to his correspondence, which claimed the mother died after Descartes's own birth. Eisenbud's (1978) emphasis is upon Descartes's investment in space and mathematics (analytic geometry) as a way to control the mother's loss at a time in the life cycle when independent locomotion through space is critical for a budding individuation. I emphasize individuation as the matrix for an experience of oneself as the originator of meaning—"*I* think; therefore *I* am." (Descartes, 1637, italics mine).

References

Abend, S. M. (1974). Problems of Identity: Theoretical and Clinical Applications. *The Psychoanalytic Quarterly,* 43, 606-637.

Abraham, K. (1924). A Short Study of the Development of the Libido Viewed in Light of Mental Disorders. In: *Selected Papers on Psychoanalysis.* London: Lowe and Beydone, 1968, 140-502.

Anthony, E. J. (1956). The Significance of Jean Piaget for Child Psychiatry. *British Journal of Medical Psychology,* 29, 20-24.

Anthony, E. J. (1958). An Experimental Approach to the Psychopathology of Childhood: Autism. *British Journal of Medical Psychology,* 31, 211-225.

Arlow, J. A. (1961). Ego Psychology and Mythology. *Journal of the American Psychoanalytic Association,* 9, 371-393.

Bach, S. (1975). Narcissism, Continuity and the Uncanny. *International Journal of Psychoanalysis*, 56, 77–86.

Bach, S. (1977) On the Narcissistic State of Consciousness. *International Journal of Psychoanalysis*, 58, 209–234.

Bach, S., and Schwartz, L. (1972). A Dream of the Marquis de Sade: Psychoanalytic Reflections on Narcissistic Trauma, Decompensation, and the Reconstitution of a Delusional Self. *Journal of the American Psychological Association,* 20, 451-475.

Bak, R. (1973). Being in Love and Object Loss. *International Journal of Psychoanalysis* , 54, 1-18.

Balint, M. (1938). Eros and Aphrodite. *International Journal of Psychoanalysis,* 19, 199-213.

Balint, M. (1948). On Genital Love. *International Journal of Psychoanalysis,* 29, 34-40.

Balint, M. (1968). *The Basic Fault. Therapeutic Aspects of Regression.* London: Tavistock.

Bell, S. (1970). The Development of a Concept of Object as Related to Infant-Mother Attachment. *Child Development,* 41, 291-311.

Beer, C. G. (1962). Incubation and Nest-Building Behaviour of Black Headed Gulls. 11: Incubation Behaviour in the Laying Period. *Behavior,* 19, 283-304.

Bergmann, M. S. (1971). Psychoanalytic Observations on the Capacity to Love. In: *Separation-Individuation. Essays in Honor of Margaret Mahler.* Ed: J. B. McDevitt and C. B. Settlege. New York: International Universities Press, 15-40.

Bergmann, M. S. (1980). On the Intrapsychic Function of Falling in Love. *The Psychoanalytic Quarterly,* 49, 56-77.

Bertalanffy, L. von (1968). *General Systems Theory.* New York, Braziller.

Bion, W. R. (1954). Notes on a Theory of Schizophrenia. *International Journal of Psychoanalysis,* 31, 113-118.

Blos, P. (1967). The Second Individuation Process of Adolescence. *The Psychoanalytic Study of the Child,* 22, 162-186. New York: International Universities Press.

Blos, P. (1968). Character Formation in Adolescence. *The Psychoanalytic Study of the Child,* 23, 245-263.

Blos, P. (1977). When and How Does Adolescence End: Structural Criteria for Adolescent Closure. In: *Adolescent Psychiatry. Developmental and Clinical Studies.* Ed: S. C. Feinstein and P. Giovacchini, 5, 5-17. New York: Jason Aronson.

Bornstein, B. (1951). On Latency. *The Psychoanalytic Study of the Child,* 6, 279-285. New York: International Universities Press.

Bouvet, M. (1958). Technical Variations and the Concept of Distance. *International Journal of Psychoanalysis,* 39, 211-221.

Bowlby, J. (1969). *Attachment and Loss.* Vol. 1, Attachment. New York: Basic Books.

Brazelton, T. B., Koslowski, B., and Main, M. (1974). The Origins of Reciprocity: The Early Mother-Infant Interaction. In: *The Effect of the Infant on its Caregiver.* Ed: M. A. Lewis and L. A. Rosenblum. New York: Wiley, 49-76.

Breuer, J., and Freud, S. (1895d). Studies on Hysteria. *Standard Edition,* Vol. 2. London: Hogarth (1955).

Brody, S. (1980). Transitional Objects: Idealization of a Phenomenon. *Psychoanalytic Quarterly,* 49, 631-667.

Buber, M. (1947). Between Man and Man. In: *Philosophy in the Twentieth Century.* Ed: W. Barrett and H. D. Aiken. Vol. 4, 688-719. New York: Random House (1962).

Burlingham, D., and Freud, A. (1942). *Young Children in War Time.* London: Allen & Union.

Calef, V., and Weinshel, E. M. (1979). The New Psychoanalysis and Psychoanalytic Revisionism. Book Review Essay on Borderline Conditions in Pathological Narcissism. *The Psychoanalytic Quarterly.* 48, 470-491.

Campbell, J. (1959). The Historical Development of Mythology. In: *Myth and Myth Making.* Ed. H. A. Murray. Boston: Beacon Press, 1960, 19-45.

Cassirer, E. (1953). *Substance and Function.* New York: Dover.

Chase, R. (1949). *Quest for Myth.* Baton Rouge: Louisiana State University Press.

Descartes, R. (1637). The Principles of Philosophy. In: *Philosophical Works of Descartes.* New York: Dover (1958).

Deutsch, H. (1942). Some Forms of Emotional Disturbance and Their Relationship to Schizophrenia. *Psychoanalytic Quarterly, 11.* 301-321.

Dewey, J. (1935). Art As Experience. In *Intelligence in the Modern World.* New York Modern Library. (1939).

Dorpat, J. L. (1979). Is Splitting a Defense? *International Review of Psychoanalysis,* 6, 105-113.

Edelheit, H. (1976). Complementarity as a Rule in Psychological Research: Jackson, Freud, and the Mind/Body Problem. *International Journal of Psychoanalysis,* 57, 23-30.

Edman, I. (1928). *Arts and The Man,* New York: Mentor (1949).

Eisenbend, J. (1978). Descartes and Shaw: Some Spatial Aspects of Object Loss. *International Review of Psychoanalysis,* 5, 285-296.

Eissler, K. R. (1950). Ego-Psychological Implications of the Psychoanalytic Treatment of Delinquents. *Psychoanalytic Study of the Child*, 5, 97–121. New York: International Universities Press.

Eissler, K. R. (1953). The Effects of the Structure of the Ego on Psychoanalytic Technique. *Journal of the American Psychoanalytic Association*, 7, 101-143.

Eissler, K. R. (1956). Panel on Problems of Identity. *Journal of the American Psychoanalytic Association*, 6, 131-142.

Eissler, K. R. (1958). Notes on Problems of Technique in the Psychoanalytic Treatment of Adolescents: With Some Remarks on Perversions. *The Psychoanalytic Study of the Child*, 13, 223-254. New York: International Universities Press.

Eliot, T. S. (1922). The Wasteland. In: *The Collected Poems and Plays of T. S. Eliot*. 1909-1950. New York: Harcourt, Brace and World (1971).

Erikson, E. (1950) *Childhood and Society*. New York: Norton.

Fenichel, O. (1945). *The Psychoanalytic Theory of Neurosis*. New York: Norton.

Ferenczi, S. (1931) Child Analysis in the Analysis of Adults. In: *The Selected Papers of Sandor Ferenczi. Problems and Methods of Psychoanalysis*. Vol. 3., 126-142. New York: Basic Books. (1955).

Fine, B. D., Joseph, E. D., and Waldhorn, H. F. (1969). The Mechanism of Denial. *Monograph 3 of the Kris Study Group of the New York Psychoanalytic Institute*. New York: International Universities Press.

Fraiberg, S. (1969). Libidinal Object Constancy and Mental Representation. *The Psychoanalytic Study of the Child*, 24, 9-47. New York: International Universities Press.

Freedman, N. (1980). On Splitting and Its Resolution. *Psychoanalysis and Contemporary Thought*, 3, 237-266. New York: International Universities Press.

Freud, A. (1936). The Ego and the Mechanisms of Defense. *The Writings of Anna Freud*. Vol. 2 (1973).

Freud, A. (1960). Discussion of Dr. John Bowlby's Paper "Grief and Mourning in Infancy." *The Psychoanalytic Study of the Child*, 15, 53-62. New York: International Universities Press.

Freud, A. (1965). *Normality and Pathology in Childhood*. New York: International Universities Press.

Freud, A. (1968). Acting out. *International Journal of Psychoanalysis*, 49, 165-178.

Freud, S. (1894a). The Neuropsychoses of Defense. *Standard Edition*, 3, 43-70. London: Hogarth (1962).

Freud, S. (1895 [1950a]). Project for a Scientific Psychology. *Standard Edition*, 1, 295-388. London: Hogarth (1966).

Freud, S. (1900a). The Interpretation of Dreams. *Standard Edition*, Vol. 4, 5. London: Hogarth (1953).

Freud, S. (1905d). Three Essays on the Theory of Sexuality. *Standard Edition*, 7, 125-243. London: Hogarth (1953).

Freud, S. (1905e). Fragment of an Analysis of a Case of Hysteria. *Standard Edition*, 7, 7-122. London: Hogarth (1953).

Freud, S. (1908b). Character and Anal Eroticism. *Standard Edition*, 9, 167-177. London: Hogarth (1959).

Freud, S. (1908e). Creative Writers and Day-Dreaming. *Standard Edition*, 9, 141-156. London: Hogarth (1959).

Freud, S. (1910h). A Special Type of Choice of Object Made by Men (Contributions to the Psychology of Love I). *Standard Edition*, 11, 165-175. London: Hogarth (1957).

Freud, S. (1911b). Formulations on the Two Principles of Mental Functioning. *Standard Edition,* 12, 215-226. London: Hogarth (1958).

Freud, S. (1911c). Psychoanalytic Notes on an Autobiographical Account of a Case of Paranoia (Dementia Paranoides). *Standard Edition,* 12, 3-84. London: Hogarth (1958).

Freud, S. (1912d). On the Universal Tendency to Debasement in the Sphere of Love (Contributions to the Psychology of Love II). *Standard Edition,* 11, 177-190. London: Hogarth (1957).

Freud, S. (1912x). Totem and Taboo. *Standard Edition,* 13, 1-164. London: Hogarth (1958).

Freud, S. (1914c). On Narcissism: An Introduction. *Standard Edition,* 14, 67-104. London: Hogarth (1957).

Freud, S. (1914g). Recollecting, Repeating and Working Through (Further Recommendations on the Technique of Psychoanalysis II). *Standard Edition,* 12, 147-159. London: Hogarth (1958).

Freud, S. (1915b). Thoughts for the Times on War and Death. *Standard Edition,* 14, 275-302. London: Hogarth (1957).

Freud, S. (1915c). Instincts and Their Vicissitudes. *Standard Edition,* 14, 111-140. London: Hogarth (1957).

Freud, S. (1915d). On Repression. Standard Edition, 14, 146-158. London: Hogarth (1958).

Freud, S. (1915e). The Unconscious. *Standard Edition,* 14, 161-261. London: Hogarth (1957).

Freud, S. (1916x). Introductory Lectures on Psychoanalysis. *Standard Edition,* 15, 3-228. London: Hogarth (1963).

Freud, S. (1917e). Mourning and Melancholia. *Standard Edition,* 14, 237-260. London: Hogarth (1957).

Freud, S. (1920g). Beyond the Pleasure Principle. *Standard Edition,* 18, 3-66. London: Hogarth (1955).

Freud, S. (1921c). Group Psychology and the Analysis of the Ego. *Standard Edition,* 18, 67-145. London: Hogarth (1955).

Freud, S. (1923b). The Ego and the Id. *Standard Edition,* 19, 3-60. London: Hogarth (1961).

Freud, S. (1923e). The Infantile Genital Organization: An Interpolation into the Theory of Sexuality. *Standard Edition,* 19, 141-148. London: Hogarth (1961).

Freud, S. (1924b). Neurosis and Psychosis. *Standard Edition,* 19, 149-156. London: Hogarth (1961).

Freud, S. (1924c). The Economic Problem of Masochism. *Standard Edition,* 19, 157-172. London: Hogarth (1961).

Freud, S. (1924e). The Loss of Reality in Neurosis and Psychosis. *Standard Edition,* 183-190. London: Hogarth (1961).

Freud, S. (1925h). Negation. *Standard Edition,* 19, 235-242. London: Hogarth (1961).

Freud, S. (1925j). Some Psychical Consequences of the Anatomical Differences Between the Sexes. *Standard Edition,* 19, 248-260. London: Hogarth (1961).

Freud, S. (1926d). Inhibitions, Symptoms and Anxiety. *Standard Edition,* 20, 77-178. London: Hogarth (1959).

Freud, S. (1927c). The Future of an Illusion. *Standard Edition,* 21, 3-58. London: Hogarth (1961).

Freud, S. (1927e). Fetishism. *Standard Edition,* 21, 149-157. London: Hogarth (1961).

Freud, S. (1930a). Civilization and Its Discontents. *Standard Edition,* 21, 64-148. London: Hogarth (1961).

Freud, S. (1933a). New Introductory Lectures on Psychoanalysis. *Standard Edition,* 27, 7-184. London: Hogarth (1964).

Freud, S. (1940a). An Outline of Psychoanalysis. *Standard Edition,* 23, 141-208. London: Hogarth (1964).

Freud, S. (1940e). Splitting of the Ego in the Process of Defense. *Standard Edition,* 23, 111-207. London: Hogarth (1964).

Fromm, E. (1956). *The Art of Loving.* New York: Harper & Row.

Frosch, J. (1970). Psychoanalytic Considerations of the Psychotic Character. *Journal of the American Psychoanalytic Association,* 18, 24-50.

Furman, R. A. (1964). Death and the Young Child. Some Preliminary Considerations. *The Psychoanalytic Study of the Child,* 19. 321-333. New York: International Universities Press.

Furth, H. G. (1964). Research with the Deaf: Implications for Language and Cognition. *Psychological Bulletin,* 62, 145-164.

Gediman, H. K. (1975). Reflections of Romanticism, Narcissism and Creativity. *Journal of The American Psychoanalytic Association,* 23, 407-423.

Gedo, J. E., and Goldberg, A. (1973). *Models of the Mind. A Psychoanalytic Theory.* Chicago: Chicago University Press.

Geleerd, E. (1965). Two Kinds of Denial: Neurotic Denial and Denial in the Service of the Need to Survive. In: *Drives, Affects, Behavior,* Vol. 2. Ed: Max Schur. New York: International Universities Press, 118-127.

Gilson, E. (1957). The Spirit of Thomism. In: *Philosophy in the Twentieth Century.* Ed: W. Barrett and H. D. Aiken. Vol. 4. New York: Random House (1962), 629-651.

Glover, E. A. (1932). A Psycho-analytic Approach to the Classification of Mental Disorders. *Journal of Mental Science,* 18, 819-842.

Goffman, E. (1959). *The Presentation of Self in Everyday Life.* New York: Doubleday Anchor Books.

Goldberg, A. (1978). *The Psychology of the Self: A Casebook.* New York: International Universities Press.

Gould, R. (1972). *Child Studies Through Fantasy. Cognitive-Affective Patterns in Development.* New York: Quadrangle Books.

Greenspan, S. I. (1979). *Intelligence and Adaptation.* Psychological Issues, Monographs 47-48.

Grubbs, J. H. (1981). A Borderline Case in Light of Piaget's Theory. In: *Three Furthur Faces of Childhood.* New York: S. P. Medical and Scientific Books, 295-305.

Hamilton, E. (1930). *The Greek Way to Western Civilization.* New York: Mentor (1948).

Hamilton, E. (1942). *Mythology. Timeless Tales of Gods and Heroes.* New York: Mentor (1953).

Hanly, C., and Masson, J. (1976). A Critical Examination of the New Narcissism. *International Journal of Psychoanalysis,* 57, 49-66.

Harlow, H. F. (1949). The Formation of Learning Sets. *Psychological Review,* 56, 51-65.

Harlow, H. F. (1958). The Nature of Love. *The American Psychologist,* 13, 673-685.

Hartmann, H. (1939). *Ego Psychology and the Problem of Adaptation.* New York: International Universities Press (1958).

Hartmann, H. (1947b). On Rational and Irrational Action. In: *Essays on Ego Psychology.* New York: International Universities Press (1964), 37-68.

Hartmann, H. (1950). Comments on the Psychoanalytic Theory of the Ego. In: *Essays on Ego Psychology.* New York: International Universities Press (1964), 113-141.

Hartmann, H. (1952). The Mutual Influences in the Development of the Ego and the Id. In: *Essays on Ego Psychology.* New York: International Universities Press (1964), 155-161.

Hartmann, H. (1953). Contribution to the Metapsychology of Schizophrenia. In: *Essays on Ego Psychology.* New York: International Universities Press (1964), 182-206.

Hartmann, H., and Lowenstein, R. M. (1962). Notes on the Super-ego. *The Psychoanalytic Study of the Child,* 17, 42-81. New York: International Universities Press.

Hartmann, H., Kris, E., and Lowenstein, R. M. (1947). Comments on the Formation of Psychic Structure. *The Psychoanalytic Study of the Child,* Vol. 2, 11-38. New York: International Universities Press.

Hemingway, E. (1921). *For Whom the Bell Tolls.* New York: Charles Scribner's Sons (1968).

Hilgard, E. R. (1948). *Theories of Learning.* New York: Appleton-Century-Crofts.

Holt, R. R. (1967). The Development of the Primary Process. In: *Motives and Thought: Psychoanalytic Essays in Honor of David Rapaport.* Psychological Issues, Monographs, 18-19, 345-383.

Jacobson, E. (1953a). The Affects and Their Pleasure-Unpleasure Qualities in Relation to the Psychic Discharge Process. In: *Drives, Affects, Behavior,* Vol. 1. Ed: R. M. Lowenstein. New York: International Universities Press, 38-66.

Jacobson, E. (1953b). Contribution to the Metapsychology of Cyclothymic Depression. In: *Affective Disorders.* Ed: P. Greenacre. New York: International Universities Press, 49-85.

Jacobson, E. (1957). Denial and Repression. In: *Depression. Comparative Studies of Normal, Neurotic, and Psychotic Conditions.* New York: International Universities Press (1971), 107-136.

Jacobson, E. (1964). *The Self and the Object World.* New York: International Universities Press.

James, W. (1890). *The Letters of William James.* Ed: H. James. Boston: Atlantic Monthly Press (1920).

Kaplan, A. (1964). *The Conduct of Inquiry.* San Francisco: Chandler Publishing Co.

Kaplan, L. J. (1972). Object Constancy in Light of Piaget's Vertical Decalage. *Bulletin of the Menninger Clinic,* 36, 322-334.

Kaplan, L. J. (1978). *Oneness and Separateness. From Infant to Individual.* New York: Simon and Schuster.

Kernberg, O. F. (1966). Structural Derivatives of Object Relationships. *International Journal of Psychoanalysis,* 47, 236-253.

Kernberg, O. F. (1974a). Contrasting Viewpoints Regarding the Nature and Psychoanalytic Treatment of Narcissistic Personalities: A Preliminary Communication. *Journal of the American Psychoanalytic Association,* 22, 255-267.

Kernberg, O. F. (1974b). Further Contributions to the Treatment of Narcissistic Personalities. *International Journal of Psychoanalysis,* 55, 215-240.

Kernberg, O. F. (1974c). Barriers to Falling and Remaining in Love. *Journal of the American Psychoanalytic Association,* 22, 486-511.

Kernberg, O. F. (1974d). Mature Love: Prerequisites and Characteristics. *Journal of the American Psychoanalytic Association,* 22, 743-768.

Kernberg, O. F. (1975a). *Borderline Conditions and Pathological Narcissism.* New York: Jason Aronson.

Kernberg, O. F. (1975b). Further Contributions to the Treatment of Narcissistic Personalities: A Reply to the Discussion by Paul H. Ornstein. *International Journal of Psychoanalysis,* 56, 245-248.

Kernberg, O. F. (1976). *Object Relations Theory and Clinical Psychoanalysis.* New York: Jason Aronson.

Kernberg, O. F. (1977). Boundaries and Structure in Love Relations. *Journal of the American Psychoanalytic Association,* 25, 81-114.

Kluckhohn, C. (1959). Recurrent Themes in Myths and Myth Making. In: *Myth and Myth Making.* Ed: H.A. Murray. Boston: Beacon Press, 1960, 46-60.

Knight, R. P. (1953). Borderline States. *Bulletin of the Menninger Clinic,* 17, 1-12.

Kohut, H. (1971) *The Analysis of the Self.* New York: International Universities Press.

Kohut, H. (1977). *The Reconstruction of the Self.* New York: International Universities Press.

Kris, E. (1952). *Psychoanalytic Explorations in Art.* New York: International Universities Press.

Lawrence, D. H. (1928). *Lady Chatterley's Lover.* New York: Grove Press (1959).

Lenneberg, E. H. (1967). *Biological Foundations of Language.* New York: Wiley.

Levin, D. C. (1969). The Self: A Contribution to Its Place in Theory and Technique. *International Journal of Psychoanalysis,* 50, 41-51.

Levinson, D. J., Darrow, C. N., Klein, E. B., Levinson, M. H., and McKee, B. (1978). *The Seasons of a Man's Life.* New York: Ballantine Books.

Levy-Bruhl, (1928). *The Soul of the Primitive.* New York: MacMillan.

Lewin, B. (1961). *The Psychoanalysis of Elation.* New York: W. W. Norstand & Co.

Lichtenberg, J. D. (1975). The Development of the Sense of Self. *Journal of the American Psychoanalytic Association,* 23, 453-484.

Lichtenberg, J. D., and Slap, J. W. (1973). Notes on the Concept of Splitting and the Defense Mechanism of Splitting of Representations. *Journal of the American Psychoanalytic Association,* 21, 772-781.

Lichtenstein, H. (1964). The Role of Narcissism in the Emergence and Maintenance of a Primary Identity. *International Journal of Psychoanalysis,* 45, 49-56.

Lichtenstein, H. (1970). Changing Implications of the Concept of Psychosexual Development. An Inquiry Concerning the Validity of Classical Psychoanalytic Assumptions Concerning Sexuality. *Journal of the American Psychoanalytic Association,* 18, 300-318.

Loewald, H. W. (1962a). Internalization, Separation, Mourning, and the Super-ego. *The Psychoanalytic Quarterly,* 31, 483-505.

Loewald, H. W. (1962b). The Super-ego and the Ego Ideal. II. Super-ego and Time. *International Journal of Psychoanalysis,* 43, 264-268.

Loewald, H. W. (1971). On Motivation and Instinct Theory. *The Psychoanalytic Study of the Child,* 26, 91-128. New York: International Universities Press.

Loewald, H. W. (1973). On Internalization. *International Journal of Psychoanalysis,* 54, 9-17.

Loewald, H. W. (1975). Psychoanalysis As an Art and the Fantasy Character of the Psychoanalytic Situation. *Journal of the American Psychoanalytic Association,* 23, 277-299.

Loewald, H. W. (1978). *Psychoanalysis and the History of the Individual.* The Freud Lectures at Yale. New Haven: Yale University Press.

Lustman, J. (1977). On Splitting. *The Psychoanalytic Study of the Child.* Vol. 32, 119-154. New York: International Universities Press.

Mahler, M. S. (1968a). *On Human Symbiosis and the Vicissitudes of Individuation.* New York: International Universities Press.

Mahler, M. S., and Kaplan, L. (1977). Development Aspects in the Assessment of Narcissistic and So-Called Borderline Personalities. In: *Borderline Personality Disorders. The Concept, the Syndrome, the Patient.* Ed: P. Hartocollis. New York: International Universities Press, 71-86.

Mahler, M. S., and McDevitt, J. R. (1968b). Adaptation and Defense in Statu Nascienti. *The Psychoanalytic Quarterly,* 37, 1-21.

Mahler, M. S., Pine, F., and Bergman, A. (1975). *The Psychological Birth of the Infant. Symbiosis and Individuation.* New York: Basic Books.

McDougall, J. (1980). *Plea for a Measure of Abnormality.* New York: International Universities Press.

Mead, G. H. (1934). *Mind, Self and Society.* Chicago: University of Chicago Press.

Metcalf, D. R., and Spitz, R. (1978). The Transitional Object: Critical Development Period and Organizer of the Psyche. In: *Between Reality and Fantasy. Transitional Objects and Phenomena.* Ed: S. A. Grolnick and L. Barkin in collaboration with W. Muensterberger. New York: Jason Aronson, 97-108.

Modell, A. (1973). Affects and Psychoanalytic Knowledge. In: *The Annual of Psychoanalysis,* 1, 117-124. New York: Quadrangle Books.

Modell, A. H. (1975). The Ego and the Id: Fifty Years Later. *International Journal of Psychoanalysis,* 50, 57-68.

Moltz, H. (1965). Contemporary Instinct Theory and Fixed Action Patterns. *Psychological Review,* 72, 27-47.

Moore, B. E. (1981). Book Review. The Psychology of the Self: A Casebook. *Journal of the American Psychological Association,* 29, 249-252.

Moore, B. E., and Fine, B. D. (1968). *A Glossary of Psychoanalytic Terms and Concepts.* New York: The American Psychoanalytic Association.

Murphy, G. (1947). *Personality. A Biosocial Approach to Origins and Structure.* New York: Harper and Brothers.

Murray, H. A. (1960). The Possible Nature of a "Mythology" To Come. In: *Myth and Myth Making.* Ed: H. A. Murray. Boston: Beacon Press, 300-352.

Nelson, K. (1974). Concept, Word and Sentence. *Psychological Review,* 81, 267-285.

Novey, S. (1955a). Some Philosophical Speculations about the Concept of the Genital Character. *International Journal of Psychoanalysis,* 36, 88-94.

Novey, S. (1955b). The Role of the Super-ego and Ego Ideal in Character Formation. *International Journal of Psychoanalysis,* 36, 254-259.

Nunberg, H. (1930). The Synthetic Function of the Ego. In: *Practice and Theory of Psychoanalysis.* New York: International Universities Press, 1960, 120-136.

Nydes, J. (1950). The Magical Experience of the Masturbatory Fantasy. *American Journal of Psychotherapy,* 4, 303-310.

Ogden, C. K., and Richards, I. A. (1923). *The Meaning of Meaning.* New York: Harcourt, Brace and World, 1946.

Ornstein, P. H. (1974). A Discussion of the Paper by Otto F. Kernberg on Further Contributions to the Treatment of Narcissistic Personalities. *International Journal of Psychoanalysis,* 55, 241-247.

Panel (1963). The Concept of Psychic Energy. Reporter: A. H. Modell. *Journal of the American Psychoanalytic Association,* 11, 605-618.

Passman, R. H., and Weisberg, P. (1975). Mothers and Blankets as Agents for Promoting Play and Exploration by Young Children in a Novel Environment. *Developmental Psychology,* 11, 170-177.

Peto, A. (1964). Variations of Archaic Thinking in Neurotics, Borderline Patients and Schizophrenics. *The Psychoanalytic Study of the Child,* 19, 73-92. New York: International Universities Press.

Piaget, J. (1924). Les Traits Principaux du Logique de l'Enfant. Cited in: J. H. Flavell, *The Developmental Psychology of Jean Piaget.* New Jersey: D. Van Nostrand (1963), 161.

Piaget, J. (1932). *The Moral Judgment of the Child.* New York: Collier (1962).

Piaget, J. (1936). *The Origins of Intelligence.* New York: International Universities Press (1952).

Piaget, J. (1941). Le Mechanisme du Dévelopment Mental et Les Lois du "Groupement" des Opérations. Cited in: J. McV. Hunt, *Intelligence and Experience.* New York: Ronald Press (1961), 203.

Piaget, J. (1945). *Play, Dreams, and Imitation in Childhood.* New York: Norton (1951).

Piaget, J. (1947). *The Psychology of Intelligence.* New Jersey: Littlefield, Adams, and Co. (1960).

Piaget, J. (1964). *Six Psychological Studies.* New York: Random House (1967).

Piaget, J. (1968). *On the Development of Memory and Identity.* Worcester, MA: Clark University Press.

Pine, F. (1979). On the Pathology of the Separation-Individuation Process As Manifested in Later Clinical Work—An Attempt at Delineation. *International Journal of Psychoanalysis,* 60, 225-242.

Pruyser, P. W. (1975). What Splits in "Splitting"? A Scrutiny of the Concept of Splitting in Psychoanalysis and Psychiatry. *Bulletin of the Menninger Clinic,* 39, 1-46.

Rapaport, D. (1957a). The Theory of Ego Autonomy: A Generalization. In: *The Collected Papers of David Rapaport.* Ed: M. M. Gill. New York: Basic Books, 1967, 722-744.

Rapaport, D. (1957b). Cognitive Structures. In: *The Collected Papers of David Rapaport.* Ed. M. M. Gill. New York: Basic Books, 1967, 631-664.

Rapaport, D. (1960). On the Psychoanalytic Theory of Motivation. In: *The Collected Papers of David Rapaport.* Ed: M. M. Gill. New York: Basic Books, 1976, 853-915.

Rapaport, D., Menninger, K., and Schafer, R. (1947). The New Role of Psychological Testing in Psychiatry. In: *The Collected Papers of David Rapaport.* Ed: M. M. Gill. New York: Basic Books, 1967, 261-275.

Rickman, J. (1928). *The Development of the Psychoanalytic Theory of the Psychosis.* London: Bailliere, Tindall, and Cox for The Institute of Psychoanalysis.

Ricoeur, P. (1970). *Freud and Philosophy.* New Haven: Yale University Press

Savitt, R. A. (1969). Transference, Somatization, and Symbiotic Need. *Journal of the American Psychoanalytic Association,* 17, 1030-1054.

Schachtel, E. G. (1947). On Memory and Childhood Amnesia. *Psychiatry,* 10, 1–26.

Schafer, R. (1968). *Aspects of Internalization.* New York: International Universities Press.

Schimeck, J. (1975). The Interpretations of the Past: Childhood Trauma, Psychical Reality, and Historical Truth. *Journal of the American Psychoanalytic Association,* 23, 845-865.

Schlam, C. C. (1976). *Cupid and Psyche. Apuleus and the Monuments.* New York: Interbook Incorporated.

Schlick, M. (1938). Meaning and Verification. In: *Philosophy in the Twentieth Century*. Vol. 3. Ed: W. Barrett and H. D. Aiken. New York: Random House, 1962, 28-51.

Schur, M. (1966). *The Id and the Regulatory Principles of Mental Functioning*. New York: International Universities Press.

Segel, N. P. (1981). Book Review. Otto Kernberg's Books. *Journal of the American Psychoanalytic Association,* 29, 221-235.

Settlage, C. F. (1977). The Psychoanalytic Understanding of Narcissistic and Borderline Personality Disorders: Advances in Development Theory. *Journal of the American Psychoanalytic Association,* 25, 805-834.

Sinclair-de-Zwart, H. (1969). Developmental Psycholinguistics. In: *Studies in Cognitive Development*. Ed: D. Elkind and J. H. Flavell. New York: Oxford Universities Press, 315-336.

Skinner, B. F. (1951). How To Teach Animals. *Scientific American,* 88, 26-29.

Sokolov, Y. N. (1963). *Perception and the Conditioned Reflex*. New York: MacMillan.

Sperling, M. (1963). Fetishism in Children. *The Psychoanalytic Quarterly,* 32, 374-392.

Spitz, R. (1962). Autoeroticism Re-examined. The Role of Early Sexual Behavior Patterns in Personality Formation. *The Psychoanalytic Study of the Child*. 17, 283-318. New York: International Universities Press.

Spock, B. (1963). The Striving for Autonomy and Regressive Object Relationships. *The Psychoanalytic Study of the Child,* 18, 361-366. New York: International Universities Press.

Stayton, R. H., Hogan, R., Ainsworth, M., and Salter, D. (1971). Infant Obedience and Maternal Behavior: The Origins of Socialization Reconsidered. *Child Development,* 42, 1057-1069.

Stein, M. (1966). Self Observation, Reality, and the Superego. In: *Psychoanalysis—A General Psychology. Essays in Honor of Heinz Hartmann*. Ed: R. M. Lowenstein, L. M. Newman, M. Schur and A. J. Solnit. New York: International Universities Press, 275-297.

Steingart, I. (1969). On Self, Character, and the Development of a Psychic Apparatus. *The Psychoanalytic Study of the Child,* 24, 271-306.

Steingart, I. (1977) A Comparative Psychopathology Approach to Language Behavior. In: *Communication Structures and Psychic Structures*. Ed: N. Freedman and S. Grand. New York: Plenum Press, 175-198.

Steingart, I., and Freedman, N. (1972). A Language Construction Approach for the Examination of Self/Object Representation in Varying Clinical States. *Psychoanalysis and Contemporary Science,* Vol. 1. Ed: R. R. Holt and E. Peterfreund. New York: International Universities Press, 132-180.

Stewart, W. A. (1970). The Split in the Ego and the Mechanism of Disavowal. *The Psychoanalytic Quarterly,* 39, 1-16.

Stolorow, R. D., and Lachmann, F. M. (1975). Early Object Loss and Denial: Developmental Considerations. *Psychoanalytic Quarterly,* 54, 596-611.

Stolorow, R. D., and Lachmann, F. M. (1978). The Developmental Prestages of Defenses: Diagnostic and Therapeutic Implications. *Psychoanalytic Quarterly,* 57, 73-102.

Stolorow, R. D., and Lachmann, F. M. (1980). *Psychoanalysis of Developmental Arrest. Theory and Treatment*. New York: International Universities Press.

Sullivan, H. S. (1940). *Conceptions of Modern Psychiatry.* Washington, D.C.: The William Alanson White Foundation.

Swinburne, A. C. (1866). Dolores. In: *The Collected Works of Algernon Charles Swinburne.* New York: Russell and Russell, 1968.

Thomas, L. (1974). *The Lives of a Cell. Notes of a Biology Watcher.* New York: Bantam Books.

Tillich, P. (1952). Courage and Individualization. In: *Philosophy in the Twentieth Century.* Vol. 4. Ed: W. Barrett and H. D. Aiken. New York: Random House, 1962, 652-687.

Tolman, E. (1932). *Purposive Behavior in Animals and Men.* New York: D. Appleton-Century.

Tolpin, M. (1972). On the Beginnings of a Cohesive Self. An Application of the Concept of Transmuting Internalization to the Study of the Transitional Object and Signal Anxiety. *The Psychoanalytic Study of the Child,* 26, 316-352. New York: International Universities Press.

Toulman, S., and Goodfield, J. (1962). *the Architecture of Matter.* New York: Harper and Row.

Trunnell, E. E., and Holt, W. E. (1974). The Concept of Denial or Disavowal. *Journal of the American Psychoanalytic Association.* 769-784.

Udry, J. R., and Morris, N. M. (1968). Distribution of Coitus in the Menstrual Cycle. *Nature,* 220, 593-596.

Vernon, M. (1967). Relationship of Language to the Thinking Process. *Archives of General Psychiatry,* 16, 325-333.

Vygotsky, L. S. (1962). *Thought and Language.* Cambridge: Massachusetts Institute Press.

Wallach, M. (1958). On Psychological Similarity. *Psychological Review,* 65, 103-116.

Werner, H., and Kaplan, B. (1963). *Symbol Formation.* New York: Wiley.

Whitehead, A. M. (1925) *Science and the Modern World.* New York: Mentor Books (1954).

Wing, L. (1972). *Autistic Children. A Guide for Parents and Professionals.* New York: Brunner/Mazel.

Winnicott, D. W. (1948). Pediatrics and Psychiatry. In: *Thought Pediatrics to Psychoanalysis.* New York: Basic Books, 1958, 157-173.

Winnicott, D. W. (1951). Playing: A Theoretical Statement. In: *Playing and Reality.* New York: Basic Books, 1971, 38-52.

Winnicott, D. W. (1953). Transitional Objects and Transitional Phenomena. In: *Playing and Reality.* New York: Basic Books, 1971, 1-25.

Winnicott, D. W. (1954a) The Depressive Position in Normal Develoment. In: *Through Pediatrics to Psychoanalysis.* New York: Basic Books, 1958, 262-277.

Winnicott, D. W. (1954b). Metapsychological and Clinical Aspects of Regression in the Clinical Set-Up. In: *Through Pediatrics to Psychoanalysis.* New York: Basic Books, 1975, 278-294.

Winnicott, D. W. (1960). Ego Distortion in Terms of the True and False Self. In: *The Maturational Processes and the Facilitating Environment.* London: Hogarth Press and the Institute of Psychoanalysis, 1965, 140-152.

Winnicott, D. W. (1963). The Mentally Ill in Your Caseload. In: *The Maturational Processes and the Facilitating Environment.* New York: International Universities Press, 1965, 217-229.

Witmer, L. (1919-22). What I Did with Don—Orthogenic Cases. XIV. Don: A Curable Case of Arrested Development Due to Fear Psychoses and the Result of Shock in a Three-Year-Old. Psychology Clinic, 1919-22, Vol. 13, 97-111. In: *Clinical Studies in Childhood Psychoses.* Ed: S. A. Szurek and I. N. Berlin. New York: Brunner/Mazel, 1973, 48-64.

Wolff, P. (1967). Cognitive Considerations for a Psychoanalytic Theory of Language Acquisition. In: *Motives and Thought: Psychoanalytic Essays in Honor of David Rapaport.* Ed: R. R. Holt. Psychological Issues, Monographs 18-19. New York: International Universities Press, 299-343.

Zilboorg, G. (1941). Ambulatory Schizophrenics. *Psychiatry,* 4, 149-155.

Index